ASPECTS OF THE HISTORY OF MEDICINE IN LATIN AMERICA

RECENT MACY PUBLICATIONS

The Impact of Health Services on Medical Education: A Global View, edited by John Z. Bowers and Elizabeth F. Purcell
New Medical Schools at Home and Abroad, edited by John Z. Bowers and Elizabeth F. Purcell
Care of the Aging, edited by Carolyn Spieler
Renal Function, edited by Gerhard H. Giebisch and Elizabeth F. Purcell

* * * * * * *

A complete catalogue of books
in print will be sent on request

Orders for all books are filled by
Independent Publishers Group
14 Vanderventer Avenue
Port Washington, New York 11050

Edited by
JOHN Z. BOWERS
and
ELIZABETH F. PURCELL

ASPECTS OF THE HISTORY OF MEDICINE IN LATIN AMERICA

Report of a Conference

JOSIAH MACY, JR. FOUNDATION
One Rockefeller Plaza, New York 10020

© 1979 Josiah Macy, Jr. Foundation
All rights reserved
Library of Congress Catalog Number: 79-91586
ISBN: 0-914362-29-1
Manufactured by World Composition Services, Inc.

CONTENTS

Foreword
John Z. Bowers / vii

Pre-Columbian Medicine:
　Its Influence on Medicine in Latin America Today
　Francisco Guerra / 1

Diseases and the Concept of Disease in Ancient Peru
　Fernando Cabieses / 16

Nutrition and Feeding Practices of the Maya in Central America
　Carlos Tejada / 54
Discussant: *E. Croft Long* / 85

Historical Synthesis of Medical Education in Mexico
　Jaime Mendiola Gomez / 88

Medicine in Colonial Brazil: An Overview
　Lycurgo de Castro Santos Filho / 97
Discussant: *Donald B. Cooper* / 108

The Teaching of Medicine In Colonial Colombia
　A. Seriano Lleras / 112

Medical Education in Latin America: A Brief Review
　Gabriel Velazquez Palau / 124

Two Footnotes to Colonial Medical History:
　The *Regimento* of Guilherme Escoph de Esens, and
　the *Erario Mineral* of Luís Gomes Ferreira, 1733 and 1735
　Charles R. Boxer / 132

The Balmis Expedition in Venezuela.
   Part II. Founding of the Central Vaccination Board, 1804
   Ricardo Archila / 142

   Documentary Appendix / 178

Participants / 183

Index/187

FOREWORD

In 1966 the Macy Foundation inaugurated programs in several Latin American countries to strengthen medical education and medical care, with special emphasis on pediatrics. As the programs developed, each year a meeting was convened of their leaders, together with other authorities in the field, at which they exchanged information about their activities. The foundation also held a meeting to discuss the use of physicians' assistants in Latin America and elsewhere, and another on Latin American schools of public health.

The history of medicine in the United States is another field in which the foundation has had a longstanding interest, and, as the Latin American pediatrics programs evolved, we became intrigued by the history of medicine in that part of the world. On 10 to 13 October 1971, therefore, a conference was held on this topic in Antigua, Guatemala.

At that conference, as reported in this volume, we learned of pre-Columbian medical practices; concepts of disease in old Peru; nutrition and feeding practices among the ancient Maya; the founding of the smallpox vaccination board in Venezuela; and other absorbing aspects of Latin American medical history, including the fact that, up until the Second World War, the medical school library holdings were almost totally dominated by French texts, such as Testut's *Anatomy*—one sign of the influence of French medicine in the Latin world; it was not until after the war that North American medical concepts became significant.

The lag between the time of the conference and publication of its proceedings must take into account the fact that further research has been done in the interim—a fact that some of the conferees wish to emphasize. Nevertheless, we hope this volume will inspire a wider interest in research in this rather neglected yet potentially fruitful field.

We are grateful for the cooperation and participation of our colleagues in Latin America, North America, and Spain.

John Z. Bowers, M.D.
President

8 November 1979

PRE-COLUMBIAN MEDICINE: ITS INFLUENCE ON MEDICINE IN LATIN AMERICA TODAY

Francisco Guerra

AMERICAN ARCHAEOLOGY

The Americas were populated as a result of successive migrations from Asia across the Bering Strait starting approximately 25,000 years ago. The arrival of the last migrants in about 5000 B.C. coincided with the development of agriculture in northern Peru and northeastern Mexico. Those 250 centuries witnessed the adaption of pre-Columbian man to an environment in which he was able to produce food and drink and develop a technology that enabled him to make tools, utensils, shelter, and clothing. He also established a family structure, political system, and religious concepts best suited to his needs. Thus by about 1000 B.C. mature civilizations existed in Mexico and Peru. At the time of the Spanish Conquest the region was populated by very primitive tribes with no knowledge of agriculture along with highly developed societies such as the Mayan, the Aztec, and the Incan.

The Maya, who settled in the highlands of Guatemala and the lowlands of Yucatan, reached their cultural summit between the fourth and tenth centuries A.D., but experienced a renaissance after the thirteenth century. They raised domestic animals and were supported by an agricultural economy based on maize and beans. Mayan society was organized around family clans in city-states, with communal sharing of land. Their religious centers such as Tikal and Chichen Itzá had great architectural beauty, featuring heavy stone structures blended with sculptural motifs. Among Mayan achievements were the exact computation of time and a hieroglyphic system.

By the middle of the thirteenth century the Aztecs had settled in the Valley of Mexico at the end of a long migration. In A.D. 1325 they founded Tenochtitlan, now Mexico City. Tenochtitlan, the largest pre-Columbian city, was superbly constructed, its pyramids with temples on top being surpassed only by the magnificence of the religious capital, Teotihuacan, a few miles to the north.

In the fifteenth century, by means of political and military alliances, the Aztecs gained control of the high plateau of Mexico, spreading their dominion to subtropical areas from whose inhabitants they extracted tribute. The arid land of the Valley of Mexico allowed only a limited agricultural economy, and the communal land was distributed among *calpulli*, family groups that in turn were integrated into an elective monarchy.

The Incas originally occupied a small area around Cuzco in the highlands of Peru; their territorial expansion early in the fifteenth century was completed when they overran the Chimu area in the north of Peru shortly before the conquest. They then proceeded to impose their language and political system on the people along the entire Pacific coast.

In the Andean highlands the Incan agricultural economy was based on potatoes; in the coastal valleys they cultivated maize. Land was communally owned, allocated to family groups (*ayllus*), and controlled by a strong administrative system responsible to a hereditary monarch with absolute power. Along the coast the Incas used clay for their buildings, including stepped pyramids resembling those of Central America; in the highlands they built with stone. The Incas had an advanced technology, particularly in metallurgy, but lacked even a pictographic calligraphy; instead they used *quipus*, colored strings with knots, with which to keep their records.

All three civilizations were flourishing at about the time the New World was discovered, but it must be kept in mind that they were the heirs to previous civilizations in the same areas: the Mochicas in northern Peru between 300 B.C. and A.D. 1000, whose agricultural system and pottery were never surpassed; and the Toltecs north of the Valley of Mexico, from 200 B.C. to almost A.D. 1000, whose technological achievements and agricultural system were inherited by the Aztecs. Medical concepts were not imported by these migrants to the New World, but, as with technological advances, were developed as the result of cumulative observations and the pre-Columbians' intellectual growth.

Unfortunately, these civilizations failed to develop the plough, wheel, quern, arch, and stringed instruments; or to invent techniques for distillation, iron smelting, and glass blowing. In many ways, although they had only a paleolithic technology they were able to solve intricate technical problems with great ingenuity in complete scientific isolation from the Old World.

DYNAMIC MEDICAL HISTORY

Medical historians have approached the study of pre-Columbian medicine[7] by analyzing the anatomical, pathological, therapeutic, and surgical tenets of these American civilizations in the light of our current knowledge of medical sciences. This approach is misleading from the ethnological point of view because it fails to assess the role of the pre-Columbian medical systems in the context of the cultural and ecological environments of these eras. A dynamic study of pre-Columbian medical concepts must examine them in relation to the physical environment and spiritual traditions of the American Indian. It must also follow their historic evolution after acculturation, the introduction of scientific medicine, and changes in urban and rural conditions. Only then can medical history demonstrate relevance in relation to the potential solution of the basic medical problems of Spanish America.

At the time of the discovery of America many different types of medical practice were identified—as many as there were ethnological groups—each one adapted to a particular civilization. Some were very primitive, almost instinctive, resembling those of the animal kingdom, as in the case of the Puelches; others involved the most elaborate clinical diagnosis, as in the case of the Aztecs. But in general they shared a similar fundamental root: disease was the punishment of supernatural powers for sins; the physician acted as an intermediary between the sick person and the supernatural powers; and treatment combined both physical and spiritual methods. E.H. Ackernecht indicates that there was a rational sequence in the concept of disease and its treatment, and that it avoided the dualism of scientific medicine with organic and psychic ailments.[1] Pre-Columbian drugs were not used for their pharmacological properties, but because they contained magic ingredients to neutralize the evil spirit of the disease.

ECOLOGICAL INFLUENCE

The American continent suffered a severe shortage of domestic animals, particularly mammals that could be used not only as sources of protein intake but as suppliers of milk for infant feeding. This had a double effect on the diets of both children and adults. In the pre-Columbian period, weaning took place very late in a child's life, at about three years of age, thus making it deeply dependent on the mother, both physically and psychologically.

The standard adult diet was based on carbohydrates—maize, beans and chili, and in certain areas potatoes and cassava. For drinking, among the Aztecs and the Maya alcoholic fermentation of the agave's sap produced *octli* or *balché*, now called *pulque*; the Mochicas and the Incas fermented maize to produce *chicha*. Both beverages had about 6 percent alcoholic content and were widely consumed because they were sometimes easier to obtain than drinking water. Inebriation was customary throughout America, although it was severely punished by the Aztecs. Children were habituated to alcohol before weaning because their mothers gave them fermented drinks early in life.

Other plants in the environment with stimulant properties have retained dietetic importance. The Tupí-Guaraní used *mate* infusion, while the Aztecs and other civilizations favored cocoa spiced with chili, vanilla, or other sweeteners. The chewing of coca leaves was customary among the Chibcha and Inca males to suppress hunger, thirst, fatigue, or mental depression. In the Caribbean and along the South American coast *cohoba* snuff was commonly used to produce hallucinations; inland the infusion of *yagé* or *ayahuasca* induced similar effects. In Central America other drugs used to produce hallucinations included *peyotl*, a cactus, *ololiuhqui*, a vine, and *teonanacatl*, a type of mushroom.[2,3]

The environment of pre-Columbian America harbored natural diseases transmitted to man by such vectors as ticks in the bushland and mosquitoes in the marshy areas. Most severe were those contagious and epidemic diseases of the tropical and subtropical areas produced by protozoaries: the trypanosomas, for example, which have been studied recently and which point up the role of triatomine as a vector.[4] In other instances, the pre-Columbian origin of epidemic disease has been questioned, as in the case of yellow fever, where the evidence has been surveyed by H.R. Carter.[5] Syphilis, and its confusion with other treponematoses, particularly yaws, has been the subject of long and bitter controversy.

CULTURAL TRENDS

The pre-Columbian communities were deeply religious, and the life of the individual was controlled from birth to death by religious rituals; in fact the existence of the American Indians had no meaning outside religion. Most of them believed in life after death, with a heaven for warriors, women who died during childbirth, and suicides. The idea of hell as a place of eternal suffering was, however, alien to them. The absence of the concept of hell as the final punishment for sinful acts was translated into cruel penalties, death in most cases, for transgressors of moral and civil laws.

The family structure and kinship system of the pre-Columbians were extremely strong, and children were raised to respect and obey their elders. Without the benefit of an ancient philosophical literary tradition, the civilization evolved into societies with moral standards similar in most respects to those of the Old World. The Aztecs, for example, had an external liturgy that resembled the sacraments of the Catholic church, with baptism, confirmation, confession, communion, marriage, and a priesthood.

The Maya and the Aztecs, particularly the latter, performed large numbers of human sacrifices as part of religious ritual. In Tenochtitlan, for example, over 20,000 victims were immolated each year, in accordance with a well-established calendar of religious feasts. The sacrifices were followed by anthropophagy. Anthropophagy was also customary among the Caribs and the Chibchas, although to them it had no religious significance. Human life in pre-Columbian America seems to have lacked the sense of transcendance found in other societies, and suicide by hanging was customary among the Inca, the Arawak, and the Maya. The Maya believed in the goddess Ixtab, who protected suicides and accompanied them to heaven.

Aztec and Mayan youths were forced to undertake painful practices of self-mutilation such as piercing limbs and ears with agave thorns, and passing a thread through a hole made in the tongue or penis. Corrective measures used by the Aztecs in raising their children included piercing the flesh with thorns, making them inhale irritating fumes, or cutting their lips for telling lies. In general the pre-Columbian man was raised with a passive attitude toward suffering and inertia in the face of travail; and he expected to die when captured in war or when he broke a tribal code.

Sexual practices differed from those of the Old World. Adultery was severely punished in all civilizations. Prostitution was common and well institutionalized, and in Mayan territory their price for intercourse was five cocoa beans. The most extensive sexual aberration was sodomy; it was customary for *bardajes*, young passive sodomites, to be used by young men before marriage. Incest was also common, particularly in the Chibcha area. Sexual aberrations differed from one area to another, however. Archaeological evidence shows that such deviations were more common among the Mochicas in northern Peru. A recent survey of erotic pottery in that area revealed that only 11 percent represented normal coitus; 31 percent were specimens of sodomy; 14 percent of fellatio; and 6 percent of bestiality and other aberrations.[6]

THE MEDICAL PROFESSION

Physicians of the pre-Columbian civilizations probably began to appear in about 500 B.C., as technology, the arts, and the hierarchies of the priesthood became well established. Their family backgrounds and social status were not, however, uniform. Among the Araucanians, for example, males with feminine behavioral traits were chosen as physicians because they were thought to be extra sensitive to human problems; in other groups, family tradition produced physicians who were trained by their elders and compelled to pass certain tests in isolation once they had decided upon a medical vocation.

In the Antilles and the North American plains the functions of the doctor were very close to or were combined with those of the priest. The medical profession branched into specialization as the pre-Columbian civilizations developed: the Incas had *soncoyoc,* common physicians who practiced medicine after going through fasts and penances; the *ichuri* who specialized in medical confessions or psychotherapy; and the *callahualas* who used medicinal plants. The Maya had a well-integrated medical profession of *ah men,* whose training included hieroglyphic writing and astrological computations. The Aztecs incorporated the Toltec heritage with knowledge obtained from conquered territories, and their physicians were highly specialized: the *ticitl* was a general practitioner knowledgeable about local diseases and their remedies; the *nahualli* used secret ingredients and horoscopes; the *tetecqui* was a surgeon who was an expert in mending bones; the *tlamatqui* was a midwife; and the *papiani* an apothecary. The Aztecs even had a *totolpixqui,* or veterinarian, expert in the care of turkeys. B. de Sahagún (circa 1565) left an excellent description of the Aztec physician:

> The physician is a curer of people, a restorer and provider of health. A good physician is a diagnostician, experienced and well-versed in the virtues of herbs, stones, trees, and roots. He is moderate in his acts; he cures people by setting bones and providing splints; he knows how to purge and to give emetics and potions; he knows how to bleed; he stitches wounds; makes incisions; and revives the sick. A bad physician is a fraud, a half-hearted worker, unskilled; a killer with his medicines because of overdosage, he worsens the condition of the sick, endangers others' lives; he pretends to be a counselor, advisor, and chaste. He bewitches, he is a sorcerer, a soothsayer, a caster of lots, he seduces women and bewitches them.[7]

Sahagún also described female doctors, and J. de Mendieta (circa 1596) indicated that men treated men and women treated women, although this does always seem to have been the case.[8]

KNOWLEDGE OF ANATOMY

Knowledge of human anatomy varied widely among different pre-Columbian civilizations. G. Olano[9] and F. Quesada[10] prepared a lexicon of Incan anatomical terms from the Quechua dictionary written by D. Gonzalez Holguin[11] in which the names of the viscera are limited and perhaps taken from organs of the guinea pig. A similar study was made of the Maya,[12] using the dictionary prepared by P. Beltran de Santa Rose, which listed about 150 terms, mostly referring to external anatomy.[13]

For the Aztecs the situation was completely different.[14] There is an abundance of names in Nahuatl—the language of the Aztecs—for the external parts of the body, but the nomenclature for viscera is poor. By combining the anatomical lexicons in Sahagún's manuscripts, which not only included descriptions of parts of the body but their appearance and texture, almost 4,000 terms were found. Unfortunately, the explanation for the Aztecs' extensive nomenclature of human anatomy lies in their practice of anthropophagy and the repeated dissections of the human body carried out by the *teopixquis*, priests who specialized in that function.

There was very limited knowledge of physiological functions, except for intestinal evacuation and the secretion of certain glands. All civilizations were aware of the pulse, but it does not follow, as F. Ocaranza once suggested,[15] that they knew about the circulation of the blood or the role of the heart. That organ did, however, play a fundamental part in religious ceremonies and was considered the center of life.

PATHOLOGY AND DIAGNOSIS

The Aztecs realized the pathological nature of some secretions, and to describe it they used the Nahuatl term for the organ or part of the body affected, together with *temalli*, purulent, or *eztli*, bloody secretion. It was universally believed that disease was a punishment for sinful acts, and it was therefore associated with the breaking of moral laws, sexual excesses and aberrations, disobedience to parents and elders, and other misdeeds. There was no all-embracing organic concept of disease, and ailments were always referred to by particular symptoms. The Aztecs identified hemorrhages, vomiting, coughing, fevers, and a great variety of diarrheas, thus demonstrating the frequency of intestinal infections due to contaminated water or spoiled food. It has been emphasized that the Maya, and to a lesser degree the Inca, identified more types of mental illness than did other civilizations: madness, frenzy, fainting spells, epilepsy, and delirium, among others.[16]

The ability of the pre-Columbian physician to integrate clinical observations with sound diagnosis appears, for example, in a description of the signs of death, *facies Hippocratica* as it is called in the classical tradition, as given in 1552 by Martin de la Cruz, the Indian physician, in *Codex Badianus*:

> The wise physician foretells from the eyes and the nostrils of the sick man whether he is going to live or die. According to his prognosis, if the eyes are bloodshot it is doubtless an indication of life; if they are pale and bloodless, recovery is uncertain. The signs of death are a certain sooty color found in the middle of the eyes, the top of the head becoming cold and contracting and depressing, the eyes darkening and losing their brightness, the nose appearing thin and pointed like a rod, the jaws becoming rigid, and the tongue cold, the teeth dusty with tartar and incapable of movement or of opening. The clenching of the teeth and the flowing of a dark or very pale blood after incision are the warnings of approaching death. In addition, the face turning livid or ashen, or its expression changing constantly. Finally, if he should roll about and unintelligible words pour from him, such as a parrot would utter . . . . [17]

Medical diagnosis was a complex procedure involving several techniques. In certain cases emphasis was placed on horoscopes and omens—the Incas and the Aztecs cast lots with grains of maize—but there was also clinical enquiry about the symptoms and the location of pain. The most important role of the physician was his precise questioning of the patient, and the first question was: "What sin have you committed?" By finding out the psychological background of the ailment he placed the patient on the road to recovery.

SURGERY AND OBSTETRICS

While surgical practice in pre-Columbian America has been highly praised, Ocaranza has demonstrated its limitations due to the lack of a proper pathological basis and inadequate control of infection.[18] Hemorrhage was avoided by compression, and examples of amputations of limbs and trepanations in mummies found in Peru indicate that surgery was performed by the control of hemorrhage and the proper suturing of the stumps, which resulted in the complete recovery of the patient.

The practice of the surgeon in Central America rested on a reasonable knowledge of external anatomy, less knowledge of internal anatomy, some idea of function, and possession of a few obsidian or flint instruments; the Incas relied on the *tumi*, a metal knife made of alloys. Surgeons used knives, saws, lancets, suture materials made of human hair or vegetable fibers, and needles made of human or animal bones or alloys. The success of a surgeon depended on his speed and dexterity in operating with the least damage to other parts of the body. These skills appear to have been well manifested in the civilizations of Central America. For example, the technique of *tlacaxipeualiztli*, or extraction of the heart via the diaphragm, was carried out in a few seconds without affecting any hard structures. Among the Incas, trepanation was extremely frequent in the treatment of head injuries, and archeological evidence demonstrates that almost 65 percent of the patients recovered. Alcoholic stupor was induced for anesthesia; in Mexico, however, a number of drugs were used to avoid pain.

Childbirth was uncomplicated, and in most pre-Columbian civilizations the mother returned to her home duties within hours after parturition. Sterility was repudiated, and barren wives were easily divorced. Midwives attended pregnancies and childbirths, and there are descriptions of how the Aztecs were able to apply external manipulation to obtain smooth and progressive dilation of the cervix so that delivery was accompanied by a minimum of trauma. N. Leon preserved a large number of very interesting records pertaining to obstetrical beliefs and practices in the Mexican area.[19]

AUTOCHTHONOUS AND EPIDEMIC DISEASES

Certain diseases were peculiar to specific pre-Columbian regions and tribes. Eskimo families experienced *piblokto*, Arctic hysteria, due to their confinement during the long winters. The Incas also described a contagious mass hysteria or dancing mania, *tanqui oncco*. But the infectious and carencial diseases prevalent in pre-Columbian civilization are of greater interest. Prior to the conquest the Incas described the *coto*, endemic goiter; *sirki*, bartonellosis or Peruvian wart; *ccara*, pinta or spirochetosis; and *uta*, cutaneous leishmaniasis; the last two diseases were also common in the Mayan area. Syphilis and yaws were extensive in the Caribbean and in continental America; despite controversies, there is anatomopathological evidence of syphilitic bone lesions in pre-Columbian Peru.[20]

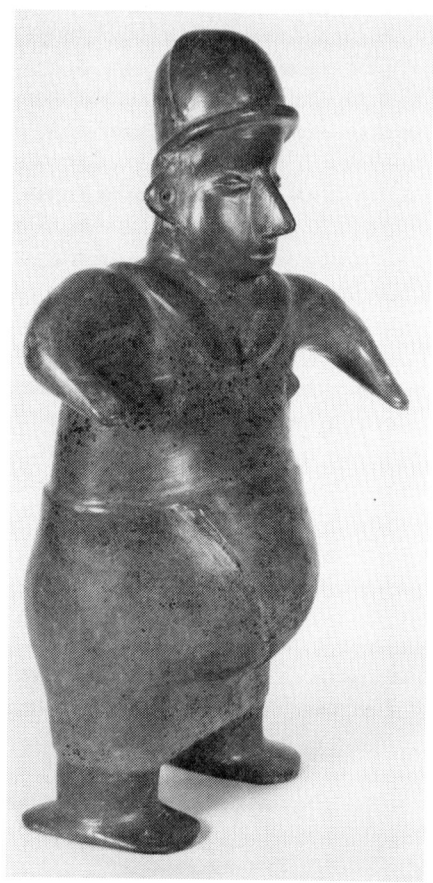

Pregnant woman (Colima culture, Western Mexico, c. B.C. 200-250 A.D.). Photograph courtesy of Manfred Waserman.

The identification of epidemic diseases, their cycles, and the degree of immunity acquired by the native population of pre-Columbian America are of considerable importance. Among the Incas, epidemics of *chavalongo*, exanthematic typhus, were common after military expeditions in the highlands. The Aztecs had a similar problem with *matlazahuatl*, typhus, which cannot always be differentiated from typhoid fever. The difficulty of identifying the Aztec *cocoliztli*—a generic name for epidemics—with yellow fever has been discussed elsewhere.[21] The Maya seem to have called it *xekik*, blood vomit, after the main symptom of the disease. A survey of certain Mayan and Mixtec codices on prognostications leaves no doubt that pre-

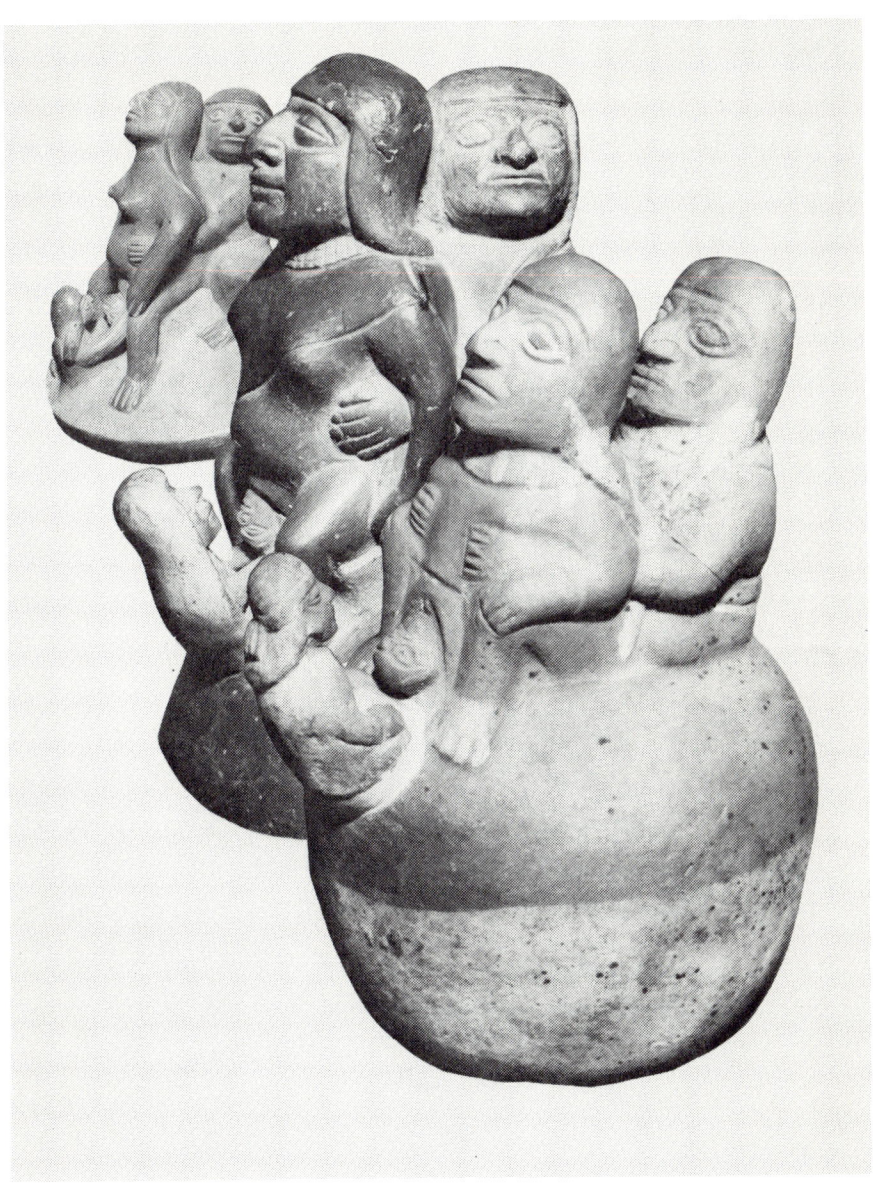

A composite photograph of Mochica women giving birth. Photograph courtesy of Fernando Cabieses.

Columbian physicians were aware that some epidemic diseases appeared in cycles.

THERAPEUTICS AND PSYCHOTHERAPY

Pre-Columbian civilizations used medicinal plants in the treatment of diseases, and learning the properties of the natural drugs was part of the training of the physician. The botanical lore has been preserved in many herbals, outstanding among which is the *Codex Badianus*: it contains illustrations of 251 plants, 185 of them reproduced in color, as well as some stones and animals used in treatment.[22] There are many other works of this type, but the survey carried out between 1570 and 1577 by F. Hernandez on more than 1,000 medicinal Mexican plants dwarfs any other study.[23] We should remember, incidentally, that coca, cinchona, *ipecacuanha*, and curare are native American plants.

It was not until recently that the curative value of the pre-Columbian practice of catharsis of the mind was fully recognized.[24] Although some early historians tried to equate it with religious confession, part of the

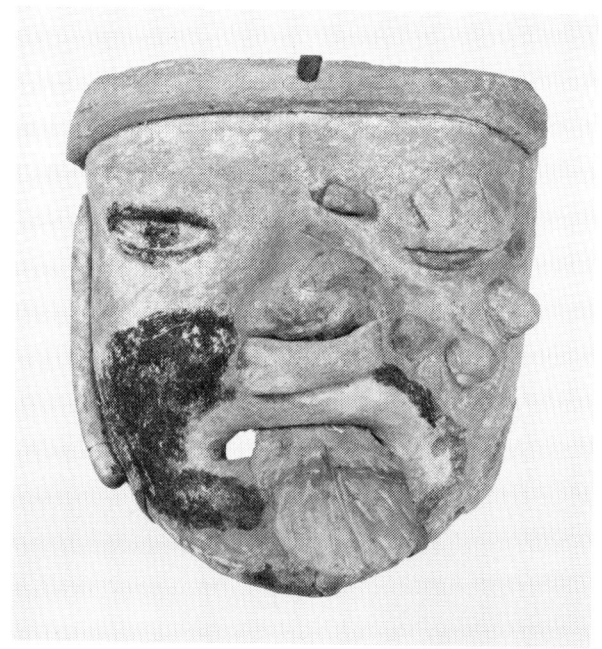

Clay mask depicting various facial lesions and tumors (Veracruz, Mexico, c. 500-900 A.D.). Photograph courtesy of the National Library of Medicine.

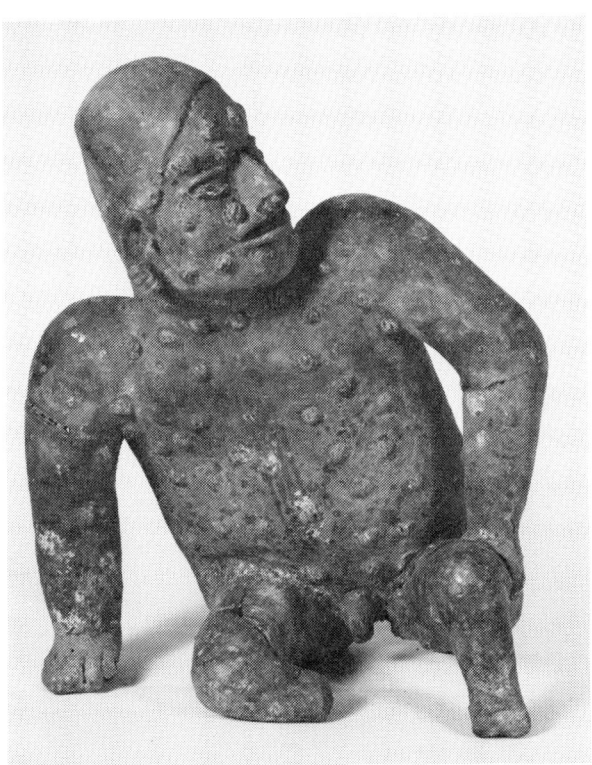

Male figure with skin lesions (yaws?) (Jalisco, Western Mexico, c. B.C. 200-250 A.D.). Photograph courtesy of the National Library of Medicine.

sacrament of penance in the Catholic church, the questioning by the physician and the confession of the patient in pre-Columbian civilizations was regarded as medical treatment for which the physician received payment. He obtained the cure by means of the therapeutic value of the word, using the same techniques as today's psychoanalyst. This practice was found among the Eskimos in the Arctic as well as among the Guaraní in South America. Among the Inca, the ritual of psychotherapy was quite elaborate. In principle, as Mendieta pointed out,[25] the physician gave the patient a preliminary examination, and if the ailment was simple he recommended the use of herbs and drugs. If the disease was serious he questioned the patient at length about his guilt until the sick person revealed every sinful act that had been bothering his conscience, sometimes for years. By the release of this psychological burden, and a ritual well adapted to the cultural trends of each civilization, the organic aspects of his ailment, if any, were ameliorated. The Incan *ichuri* specialized in such treatments, which were divided into hierarchies of minor to severe transgressions. They completed the treatment and the psychological transfer by ordering the patient to wash in running water. The Aztec *ticitl* and the Mayan *ah men* used similar methods of spiritual catharsis, by which they revealed, in particular, a patient's sexual aberrations; after confession the patient went to the *temazcalli*, steam bath, to cleanse his body.

THE PRE-COLUMBIAN LEGACY

Large masses of the population of Spanish America, in both rural and urban areas, have retained the traditional pre-Columbian systems of medicine in the treatment of organic and mental illness. Medicinal plants, bone manipulation, and religious rituals are still used in addition to, or instead of, modern scientific medicine.

These systems are successful in the majority of cases because the self-curative powers of nature are integrated with curative concepts well adapted to the minds and to the cultural and physical environments of the people. The pharmacological activity of most medicinal plants has seldom been confirmed, but the magic element is there, and the traditional position of trust the native physician holds in the community has remained unchanged. He and the priest still control the practice of psychotherapy; their influence cannot be ignored because it has its roots in the ancestral religion of pre-Columbian life.

Pre-Columbian civilizations in their process of adaptation and survival reached a balance with their own natural diseases, vectors, reservoirs, and epidemic cycles. This could explain their commensalism with respect to certain protozoic infections.

NOTES

1. E.H. Ackernecht, "Natural Diseases and Rational Treatment in Primitive Medicine," *Bulletin of the History of Medicine* 19 (1946): 467-97.
2. F. Guerra, "Mexican Phantastica," *British Journal of Addiction* 62 (1967): 171-87.
3. C. Coury and M.D. Grmek, *La médecine de l'Amerique precolombienne* (Paris: Ed. Roger Dacosta, 1969).
4. F. Guerra, "American Trypanosomiasis. A Historical and a Human Lesson," *Journal of Tropical Medicine and Hygiene* 73 (1970): 83-118.
5. H.R. Carter, *Yellow Fever: An Epidemiological and Historical Study of Its Place and Origin* (Baltimore: Williams & Wilkins, 1931).
6. F. Guerra, *The Pre-Columbian Mind* (London: Seminar Press, 1971).
7. B. de Sahagún, *História General de las Cosas de Nueva España* (México: P. Robredo, 1938).

8. J. de Mendieta, *História Eclesiástica Indiana* (Mexico: F. Díaz de León and S. White, 1870).

9. G. Olano, "Conocimientos Anatómicos de los Antiguos Peruanos," *Crónical Médica* (Lima) 26 (1919): 78-86.

10. F. Quesada, "La Anatomía en el Perú Durante el Imperio de los Incas," *Crónical Médica* (Lima) 26 (1919): 415-29.

11. D. Gonzalez Holguin, *Grammatica y Arte Nueva de la Lengua General de todo el Perú Lllamada Lengua Quichua o Lengua del Inca* (Lima: F. del Canto, 1607).

12. F. Guerra, "Maya Medicine," *Medical History* 8 (1964): 31-43.

13. P. Beltrán de Santa Rosa, *Arte del Idioma Maya Reducido a Succintas Reglas y Semilexicon Yucateco* (Mexico: Vda. de J.B. Hogal, 1746).

14. F. Guerra, "Aztec Medicine," *Medical History* 10 (1966): 315-38.

15. F. Ocaranza, *La Cirgía en el Anahuac Durante le Época pre Cortesiana* (México: Ed. Laboratories Midy, 1936).

16. Guerra, "Maya Medicine" (See note 12).

17. M. de la Cruz, *Codex Badianus* (1552), cited in *Libellus de Medicinalibus Indorum Herbis*, ed. F. Guerra (Mexico: Vargas Rea and Diarios Español, 1952).

18. Ocaranza, *La Cirugía en el Anahuac* (See note 15).

19. N. León, *La Obstetricia en Mexico* (Mexico: F. Díaz de León, 1910).

20. J.C. Tello and H.C. Williams, "An Ancient Syphilitic Skull from Paracas in Peru," *Annals of Medical History*, n.s., 2 (1930): 515-29.

21. F. Guerra, *La Medicina Precolombina* (Barcelona: Salvat Ed., 1971).

22. Cruz, *Codex Badianus* (see note 17).

23. F. Hernandez, *Rerum Medicarum Novae Hispaniae Thesaurus* (Rome: V. Mascardi, 1628).

24. Guerra, *Pre-Columbian Mind* (See note 6).

25. Mendieta, *História Eclesiástica* (See note 8).

DISEASES AND THE CONCEPT OF DISEASE IN ANCIENT PERU

Fernando Cabieses

Disease is a reaction of the body to an assault from the environment, both internal and external. Victory, defeat, or continued struggle follow as a result of this imbalance between the body and its environment. The objective signs of disease are produced in a complicated convergence of equations whereby the person's biological constants, psychological reactions, and cultural tendencies come into conflict with the offensive agent, whether it be a germ, a physical, chemical, or psychological trauma, or a congenital defect.

Following this line of logic we should not be surprised by the endless discussions of the history of disease. Man has changed and continues to change; germs have changed and continue to change. Because of these two biological facts, diseases are also changing and will continue to change in both their objective signs and subjective expressions.

When we read the clinical description of syphilis written by Fracastorius in 1530, for example, it is difficult to recognize the disease that now goes under that name. Nevertheless, both groups of symptoms—those of the Rennaissance era and those of the Atomic Age—are the results of conflict between man and the pale spirochete. This is not because man has conquered the disease with arsenic compounds or antibiotics during the last fifty years: even when Ehrlich developed his magic bullet—the arsenic compound that constituted the first radical cure for syphilis in the last century—the symptomatology of the disease had already changed.

The same can be said of leprosy. Much of the awe that this disease inspired originated from terrifying descriptions found in the Bible and in writings during the Middle Ages. But even before the advent of modern drugs and the development of our present knowledge of leprosy it had ceased to be the traditional dominant bacterial disease of Europe, perhaps because of man's adaptation or partial immunization to it.

Countless examples may be cited to illustrate why it is impossible to reach an exact diagnosis of a "disease" from the description of the plagues and epidemics of medieval Europe. Even in this century it is difficult for us to recognize the relatively benign influenza of our day from the alarming descriptions of the havoc it caused in 1918. Much less can medical historians today identify with any degree of accuracy the etiology of the Black Death of the fourteenth century, or the cause of epidemics so well described by Hippocrates four centuries before Christ.

We must therefore establish definite limits to identification of diseases described by chroniclers who visited Peru in the sixteenth century. Even realistic presentations of anatomical lesions shown in the ceramic figures of some pre-Columbian cultures must be studied with a critical eye.

Infections and psychosomatic diseases clearly belong in the category of pathology in evolution. Congenital, traumatic, or metabolic diseases, on the other hand, since they are caused by factors less inclined to rapid change, have much more stable characteristics. Furthermore, symptoms such as pain, fever, coughs, diarrhea, convulsions, loss of weight, inflammation, suppuration, and anatomical deformities constitute scarcely variable elements to which we can revert to describe the reactions of ancient man to certain diseases.

Thus, while we do make advances, progress is limited because we cannot accurately identify a current disease on the basis of symptoms that occurred many centuries ago. If we do not work within this limitation, we may be forced into a totally allegorical paleopathology. A fractured bone; a congenitally defective hip; an osteoarthritic spine; a mummified scalp infested with lice; cholesterol deposits in the arteries of a mummy; a harelip depicted in a ceramic head—all these diagnostic elements are incontrovertible. But what seems to be a skin rash in a ceramic figure, an area of erosion in a bone, or the possible but ambiguous proof of intercranial pressure in an ancient skull, leave much to be desired as useful factors on which to base an accurate diagnosis. Descriptions of a fever, a headache, general indisposition, joint pains, a cough, and a skin rash may be accepted at face value if they come from a trustworthy source. But the integration of this group of symptoms with the diagnosis of a disease known to modern medicine is plagued with uncertainty and danger. Such a chain of clinical data might have occurred after an infectious or toxic process, not necessarily after smallpox or other eruptive diseases.

While we are at a disadvantage, the identification of diseases that occurred in ancient Peru might constitute a productive way to study the medicine practiced in that culture. This road has in fact been followed fruitfully by researchers such as A. Hrdlicka,[1] R. Moodie,[2-4] H.U. Williams,[5] J.C. Tello,[6] P. Weiss,[7-9] J.B. Lastres,[10,11] O. Dabbert,[12] and Urteaga Ballón.

As shown in their various aspects in ceramics, the names of diseases were rooted in Indian vocabularies of the sixteenth century. We will therefore mention language when it might help to illustrate the present discourse.

The word *oncoy*, or *unccoy*, for example, means a general clinical process equivalent to our concept of "disease" and is found in many medical terms of ancient Peru. The symptom itself frequently indicated the disease, such as Quechuan words that translate into fever, headache, cough, urinary difficulties, loss of weight, and bloody evacuation. Other Quechuan words identify clinical entities as we know them today; goiter, epilepsy, madness, warts, and asthma, for example. Among this group of medical terms is found the name of a disease such as *uta*, which, because of its peculiarity to certain areas and the impossibility of translating it into Spanish, has been adopted by modern medical language.

DISORDERS OF THE BONE

Ancient Peruvians undoubtedly knew the symptoms of rheumatoid arthritis, but we are not sure if they recognized it as a specific clinical entity. Mummies and skeletons found in archaeological areas show clear evidence of this disease, which is also found in the mummies of other ancient races of the world. The Quechuan term *tullu-oncoyniuoc* (*tullu* meaning bone) translates as a painful disease of the bones. It is no better or worse a term than rheumatism, which we use to refer to an inflammation or an unspecified flux in a specific area of the body.

In Peruvian museums there are vertebrae and long and short bones that show typically rheumatic injuries that probably caused the same degree of pain they cause modern man. At the time he was searching for these types of injuries, Hrdlicka found a special type of deforming arthritis of the hip that occurred only in adolescents, and that had a progressive, usually unilateral, development.[13] This type of arthritis caused a shortening of the neck and a flattening of the head of the femur, rugosity, and a flattening of the hip joint. While very few studies have been made of Hrdlicka's findings, it is evident that this disease cannot be accepted as typical rheumatoid arthritis. He also found minor lesions in other joints

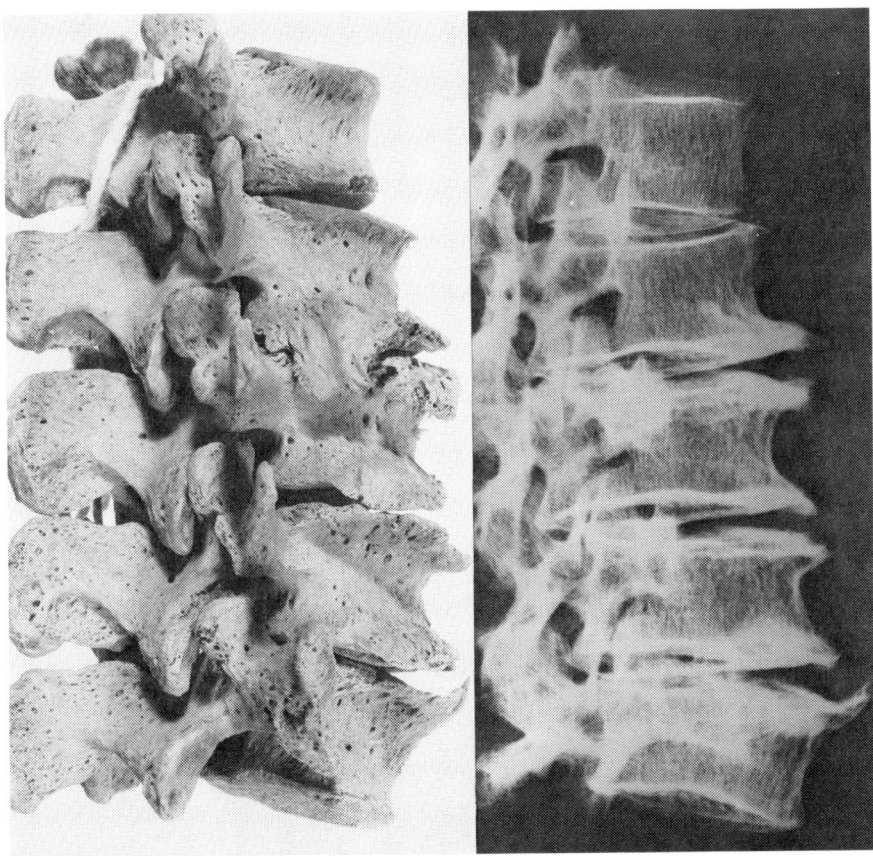

Part of the spinal column of a Peruvian mummy showing the typical findings of spondyloarthrosis (Chancay culture, c. 1300 A.D.).*

coinciding with the disturbance of the hip, but this has not been substantiated by other researchers. Since this disorder had never been found in any other ancient culture, it was very difficult to identify it with a modern disease. According to Hrdlicka it occurred with greater frequency along the coast than in mountains. Modern experts tend to classify the disease as the result of a congenital luxation, or a condition of the hip known as Perthes-Calvét disease, the exact cause of which is not known.

---

* All photographs in this chapter are courtesy of Dr. Cabieses.

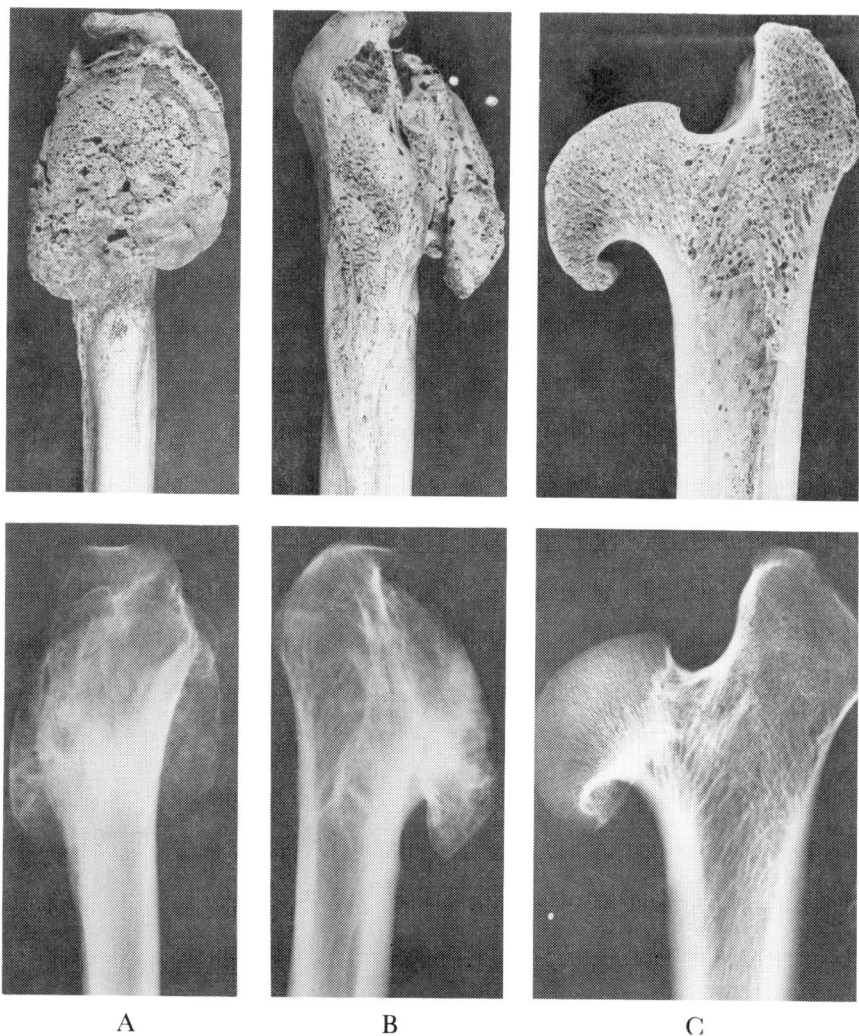

A   B   C

Two cases of a degenerative condition of the head of the femur (Mochica culture, c. 800 A.D. A and B represent very pronounced cases; C is a mild case (see text).

FEVERS

The word *rupha* means fever. In ancient vocabularies we find the term, *chayapuc-rupha-onccoy*, a disease characterized by periodic fevers, probably identified as malaria. In modern Quechuan Cuzqueño dialect, malaria is called *chucchu*, which means chill. It is believed that this disease existed in Peruvian coastal valleys since time immemorial, and some descriptions indicate that malaria was one of the greatest enemies of the Incan armies in the era of Pachacute. From the descriptions found in Spanish chronicles we have no reason to doubt that it was also a most serious hazard to Pizarro's invading armies.[14]

CANCER

We can confirm signs of primary or secondary malignant tumors in bones found in pre-Columbian cemeteries in Peru. Ceramic pieces also provide evidence that cancer was present in Peru at that time.

In ancient Quechua the term *yzco-unccoy*, or *yzuni-onccoy*, translates as cancerous. A correct translation of this term, however, must take into

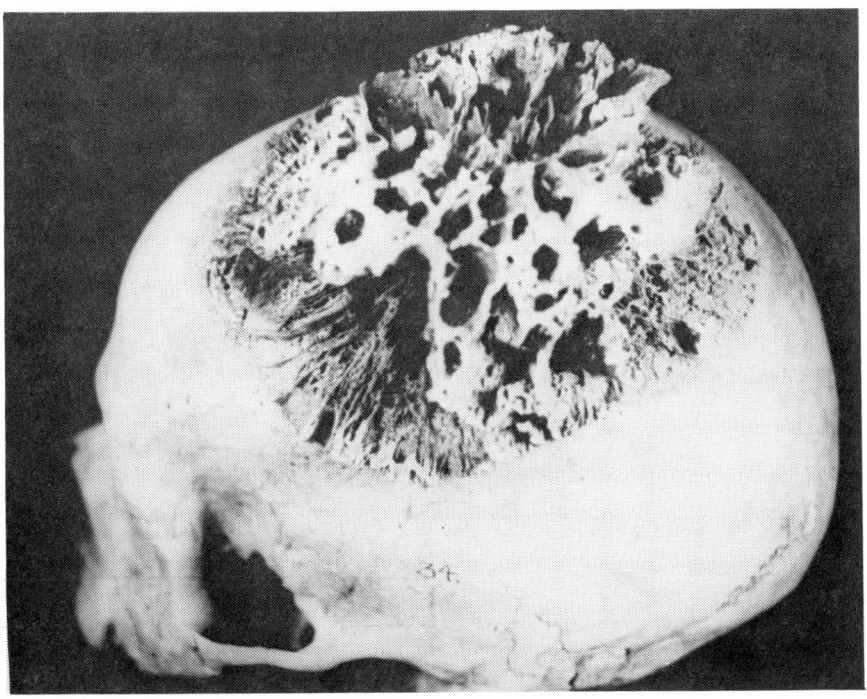

Large tumor of the skull, probably an outsized meningeoma. Skull was found in a burial cave near Macchu-Picchu by the Bingham expedition in 1913.

account that diagnosis at that time was limited to a gross anatomical examination, and that probably neither ancient Peruvians nor their Spanish translators could differentiate cancer from gangrenous tissue. Since *yzmuni* means to rot or to become putrid, the term simply meant a rotting disease—the modern word cancer is not much more descriptive than that. The conquistadores described the unsightly ulcers produced by an infectious process as cancer, and Fray Antonio de la Calancha stated in his excellent description of Incan medicine that Indian healers used an herb and the powder from a small seashell to make a paste with which to treat cancer.

SYPHILIS

The great Peruvian physician and archaeologist, Julio Tello, believed that syphilis, apparently identified by the Quechuan word *huanti*, had left its imprint on the bones of ancient Peruvians.[15] The origin of the disease in the New World, and its possible importation from America to Europe, has caused endless scientific controversies. The great majority of researchers favor America as the source, based on the theory that its appearance in Europe began when Columbus's sailors returned from Hispaniola with so-called *Napolitana* or French disease. It was around that time that Antonio de Herrera, another chronicler, wrote that one of the most common diseases in South America was the *bubas*, a seemingly venereal ailment that produced genital secretions and that was treated successfully with sarsaparilla and guaiacum.[16] Another chronicler, Francisco López de Gomara, repeatedly stated that all Peruvians suffered from the *bubas*, and that Spaniards who had who had sexual intercourse with Indian women became infected.[17]

That is very interesting, but we cannot confirm that the Spaniards equated syphilis with *bubas*. Venereal diseases had not been studied enough at that time, and the symptoms covered not only syphilis and gonorrhea, but the "third" venereal disease—Favre's disease, or lymphogranuloma—which bears more of a resemblance to the *bubas*. The clinical manifestations of syphilis have changed so much, however, that efforts to identify it from early descriptions meet with serious obstacles.

As for anatomical evidence, all we have are the imprints on bones recovered from Peruvian cemeteries, which show a special type of deformation of the surface of the bone that some investigators doubt are absolutely specific for syphilis. Many experts believe the same type of scar may have been caused by other chronic inflammatory diseases of the bone.

Several years ago, prehistoric bones discovered in the United States showed this type of pathology. Tello and H. Williams attribute considerable importance to the famous syphilitic skull from Paracas, and detailed descriptions and excellent photographs leave little doubt as to the diagnosis.[18] Williams is totally convinced of the existence of syphilis in pre-Columbian America, based on his study of the Pecos skull described by A.V. Kidder and E. Hooton,[19] the skull from Rio Negro, and others from Paracas. G.F. Eaton and G. McCurdy, the anthropologists who accompanied Hiram Bingham in the discovery of Macchu Picchu, also described apparently syphilitic bones in the archaelogical area around Cuzco,[20,21] and Peter Weiss found similar evidence in the Huaura culture of the Peruvian coast.[22]

Although the work of all these researchers seems to prove the prehistoric antiquity of syphilis in America, there is equally trustworthy information that this disease—or one that left similar marks on the bones—was present in Europe before Columbus arrived in Hispaniola. Investigations carried out by several other workers lead us to believe that syphilis has in fact existed throughout the world since time immemorial.

In all probability, therefore, Columbus's sailors did not carry a new germ back to Europe, but, rather, a special strain of spirochete, which although apparently well tolerated by the Indians was severely damaging to the white race on the old continent.

UTA

Uta, a special type of American leishmaniasis, is a very old Peruvian disease. It produces mutilating ulcers on the nose and lips that are very difficult to cure, and although they eventually do heal they leave severe scars. Mention of this disease, called the "cancer of the Andes" by the Spaniards, dates back to the beginning of the conquest and has appeared repeatedly during the ensuing centuries. The *uta* is found on both sides of the Andes—in the humid ravines of the Pacific slopes, and in the warm valleys of the jungle.

Perhaps the first to mention *uta* was Pedro Pizarro, who in about 1537 wrote that those who entered the jungle contracted a "disease of the nose" very similar to leprosy for which there was no cure, although there were Indian remedies that alleviated it.[23] F. de Santillan, another writer of the time, wrote of the frequency with which Indians who went into the jungle to cultivate coca contracted this disease;[24] and Fray Rodrigo Loayza also mentioned it by the name *andeongo* (*anti-onccoy*), a disease of the Andes that "corrodes the nose."[25]

Uta has caused heated controversies among modern paleopathologists. When the Anthropological Society of Berlin met in 1895, a spectacular scientific duel took place among the participants. The stir originated in relation to a group of ceramic pieces of the Mochica culture depicting individuals whose noses and upper lips were mutilated. A. Ashmead, the American anthropologist, maintained in a well-documented speech that the injuries were caused by leprosy. On the other hand, Rudolph Virchow, the renowned Viennese pathologist, presented his convincing opinion that the lesions were the results of syphilis. After many hours of discussion the matter was still not resolved, and everyone left Berlin without having changed his opinion.

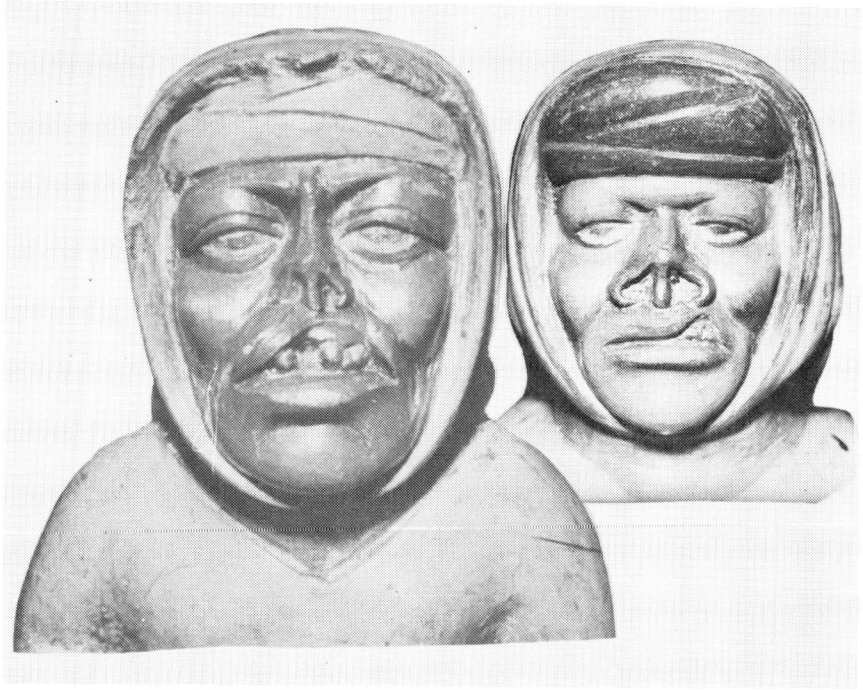

Type of lesion, probably punitive mutilation, shown frequently in ceramic figures of the Mochica culture. Such representations have given rise to lengthy controversies (see text).

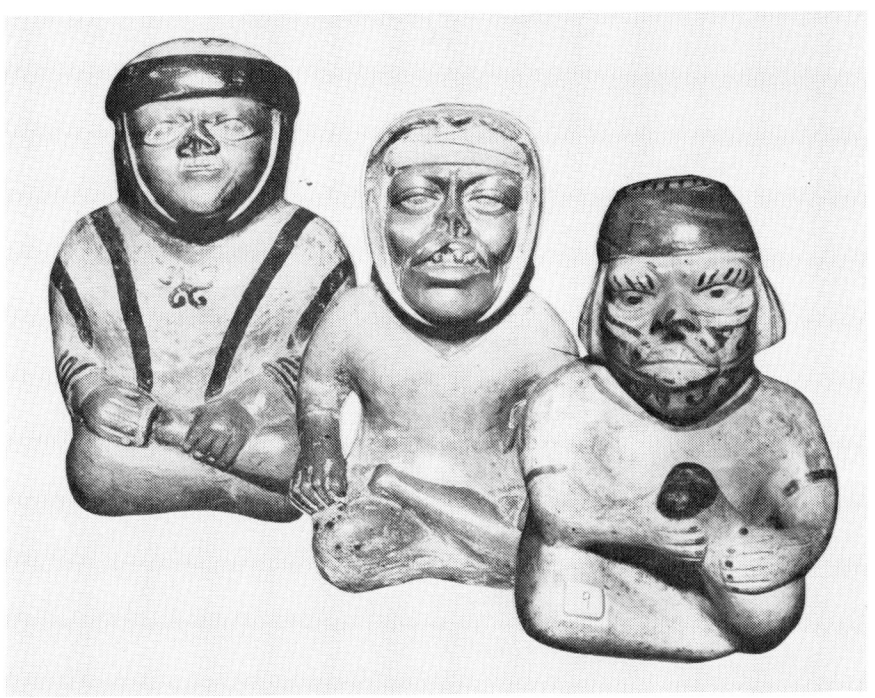

Lesions, probably punitive mutilations. Notice the amputation of the foot. These figures are arranged to show three stages of rehabilitation, the final one exhibiting the use of a prosthetic cap on the stump (Mochica culture).

Several years later, at the International Congress on Leprosy, again in Berlin, Polakowski gave a mortal blow to Ashmead's theories. Having obtained considerable data from Carrasquilla in Colombia, Polakowski called attention to the fact that no Spanish or Indian chronicles mentioned the presence of leprosy on the American continent before the conquest. If leprosy had existed it would certainly not have escaped the observation of the Spanish, who were painfully familiar with this terrible disease, which constituted a scourge in medieval Europe. After reviewing all the ancient texts, Polakowski and Carrasquilla proposed that the injuries shown in the Mochica pieces were probably due to punitive mutilation rather than to any type of disease.

A month later another meeting of the Anthropological Society of Berlin took place with the participation of famous Americanists such as

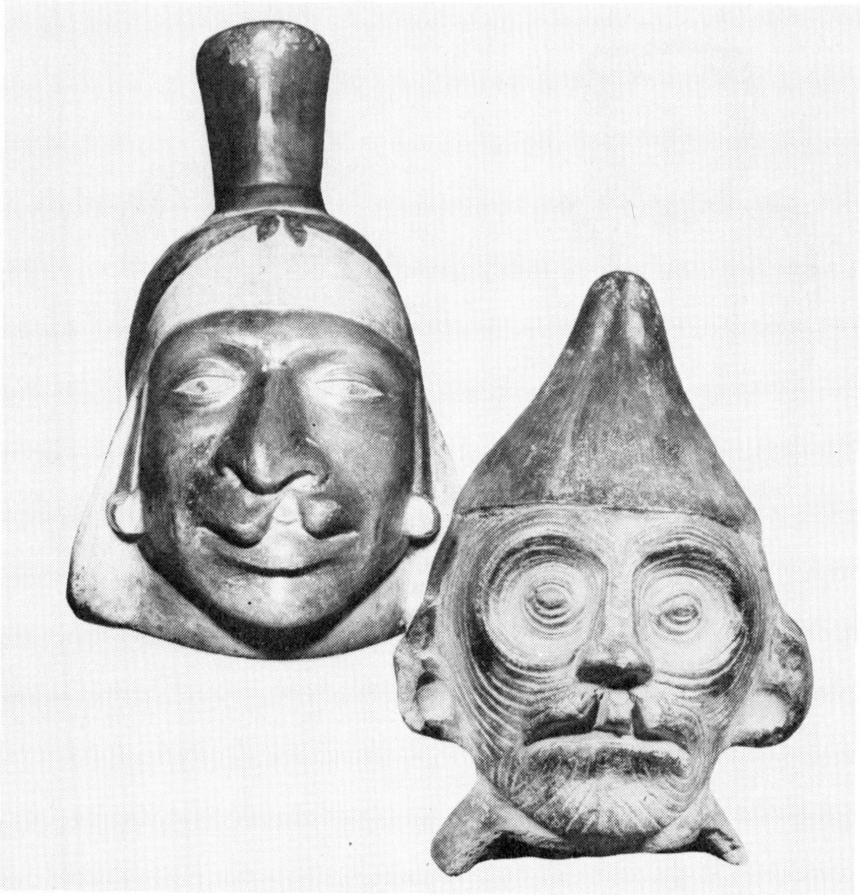

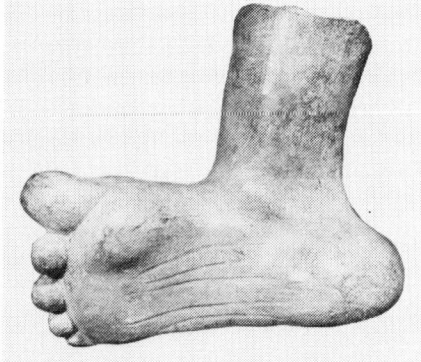

Above: two ceramic vessels depicting persons with harelips. The man in the foreground shows ritual scars on the face (Chimu culture); the one in the background is from the Mochica culture.
Left: a clubfoot (Mochica culture).

Midendorf, Stubel, Von Den Steinen, Seler, and Jiménez de la Espada. Again the concept of *uta* as the inspiration of the Mochica artists was introduced, and Ashmead summarized the discussions by pointing out that what the ceramics represented could have had many origins—punitive mutilation, *uta*, tuberculosis, leprosy, or syphilis. The controversy still continues.

If the present author had to give a definite opinion he would favor punitive mutilations: leprosy did not exist in Peru before the arrival of the Spaniards; even at that time syphilis very rarely produced such serious injuries; and *uta* destroys the septum, leaving only a hole where the nostrils used to be, and, furthermore, it was rarely found in the areas where the Mochicas lived. With respect to mutilation, the chronicles are full of precise descriptions of this type of punishment, as well as of the amputation of legs and arms, disfigurements that are present in almost all ceramic pieces that show facial injuries.

This might be a wrong interpretation, and those who favor *uta* as the culprit may be right, at least in some instances. But a dogmatic attitude toward the interpretation of signs and the description of ancient diseases has never been so out of place, and this review may serve as a word of warning to all who are interested in paleopathology.

ENDOCRINOLOGICAL DISORDERS

Endocrinological disorders in ancient Peru are well represented in ceramic pieces. We see evidence of obesity and dwarfism, for example, and some skulls show the typical characteristics of acromegaly, a variety of gigantism produced by a pituitary tumor that causes overproduction of growth hormones. The Quechua had many terms for such disorders, although there is no indication that they interpreted them as true diseases. In many primitive and developed cultures this type of symptomatology is considered not so much pathological as individual characteristics compatible with health. F. Huamán-Poma gives an example when he refers to Capac-Umi-Tallana, a noblewoman from Collasuyo, "having once been a great beauty, she gained so much weight she became as ugly as all her relatives, who are generally fat, lazy, weak, inefficient, and shy."[26]

CONGENITAL MALFORMATIONS

Ancient Peruvian ceramic craftsmen depicted congenital malformations, believing they were produced by a divine act. It is difficult to overlook the excellent representations of harelip, club foot (*pie-bot*), and other deformities. A famous ceramic piece first reproduced by Moodie was interpreted by this author as representing a case of *gondou*, another type of leishmaniasis frequently seen in Africa, but never observed in Peru.[27] We believe this representation in Peruvian ceramics probably showed a cranionasal meningocele, a congenital malformation of the anterior part of the base of the skull that produces a tumor in the root of the nose.

Malformations of the spinal cord are to be found in skeletons in old Peruvian cemeteries. They are not very common, however, and because similar specimens are frequently found in other parts of the world, those in Peru fall more within the frame of medical curiosities than interesting discoveries. Were it not for very obvious malformation that produces a shortening or deviation of the spine, this type of pathology would probably have been overlooked by both artists and scientists. We have not seen an authentic ceramic representation of a spinal meningocele or of any other case, such as spina bifida, that could be clinically diagnosed.

TUBERCULOSIS

There is evidence that tuberculosis existed in pre-Columbian Peru. In the Quechuan vocabulary there are terms such as *chhaque-unccoy*, *chullu-unccoy*, and *sucyay-unccoy*, meaning the presence of a disease that causes loss of weight and atrophy, which may be accompanied by a cough, and at times by hemoptysis, "blood that comes from the veins of the chest." One must not be misled by some investigators who theorize that tuberculosis occurred infrequently in ancient Peru because "misery was not known in their social system." Many other factors certainly contributed to the development of tuberculosis; chroniclers described long periods of famine or local plagues, for example. From the behavior of the tuberculosis bacillus in historical times it can be said with some assurance that cases of tuberculosis were more frequent in the coastal valleys than in the mountains. J.E. García Frías has stated that he found radiological proof of tuberculosis in the lungs and spinal cord of pre-Columbian mummies around the Jauja area.[28]

Ceramic representations and the drawings of Huamán-Poma demonstrate the typical appearance of individuals suffering from tuberculosis of the spinal column; in some mummies found in the coastal region the skeletons show clear evidence of this disease.

Other disorders of the respiratory system appeared in old Quechuan vocabularies. We find words that identified asthma, (*karcay-unccoy*), pneumonia, (*zamaypiti*), and the common cold, (*chullicuni*), demonstrating that ancient Peruvians classified diseases as clinical entities, going a step further

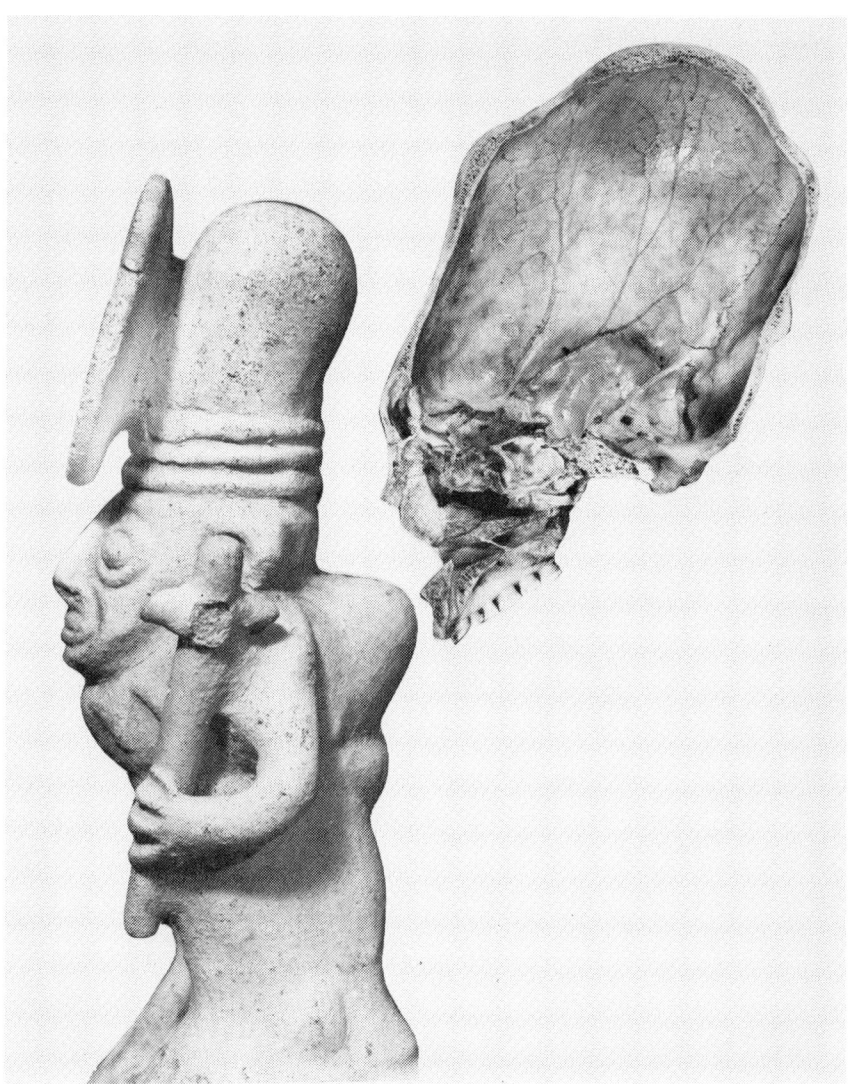

Besides depicting a probable case of tuberculosis of the spine, this Chancay figurine shows the cranial deformation produced artificially in early childhood. Skull to the right shows similar deformation.

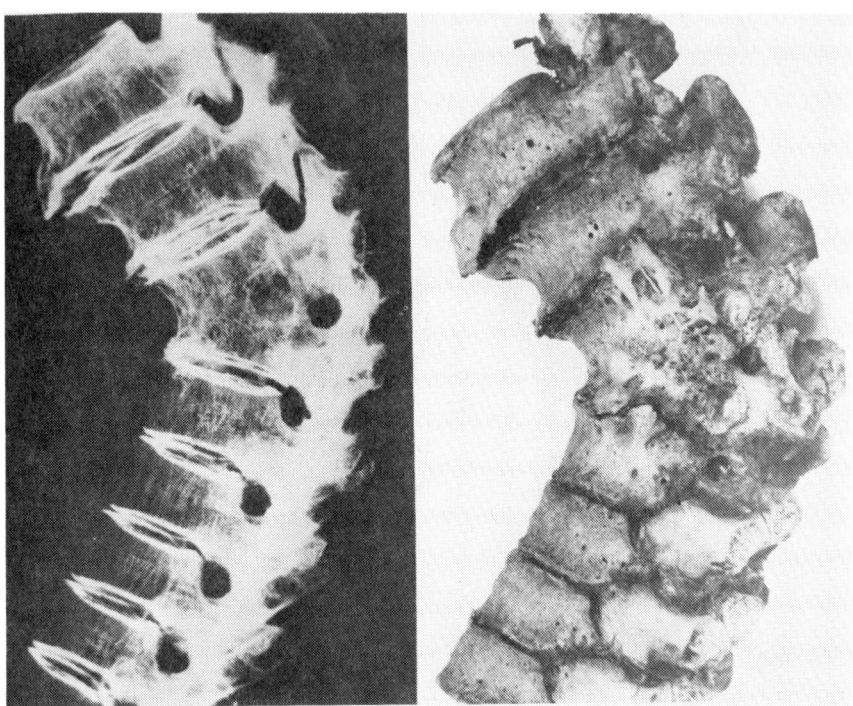

Spinal column showing the results of healed tuberculosis of the vertebral bodies (Chancay culture).

than the primitive concept of identifying them merely on the basis of their symptomatologies.

PERUVIAN VERRUGA

Another prevalent disease in pre-Columbian Peru was so-called Peruvian verruga (Oroya fever, or Carrión's disease), which has never been found outside the Inca area. It is caused by *Bartonella bacilliformis*, which is transmitted by a sandfly found in midaltitude Andean valleys. Peruvian verruga is a serious, often fatal, ailment characterized by high fever, rapid weakening, and anemia, followed by the appearance of a skin rash of a warty type that generally marks the crisis of the disease. It is probably identified in Quechuan by the word *sirki*, which differs from *ticti*, the common wart, and from *kcepo*, the boil.

DISEASES IN ANCIENT PERU 31

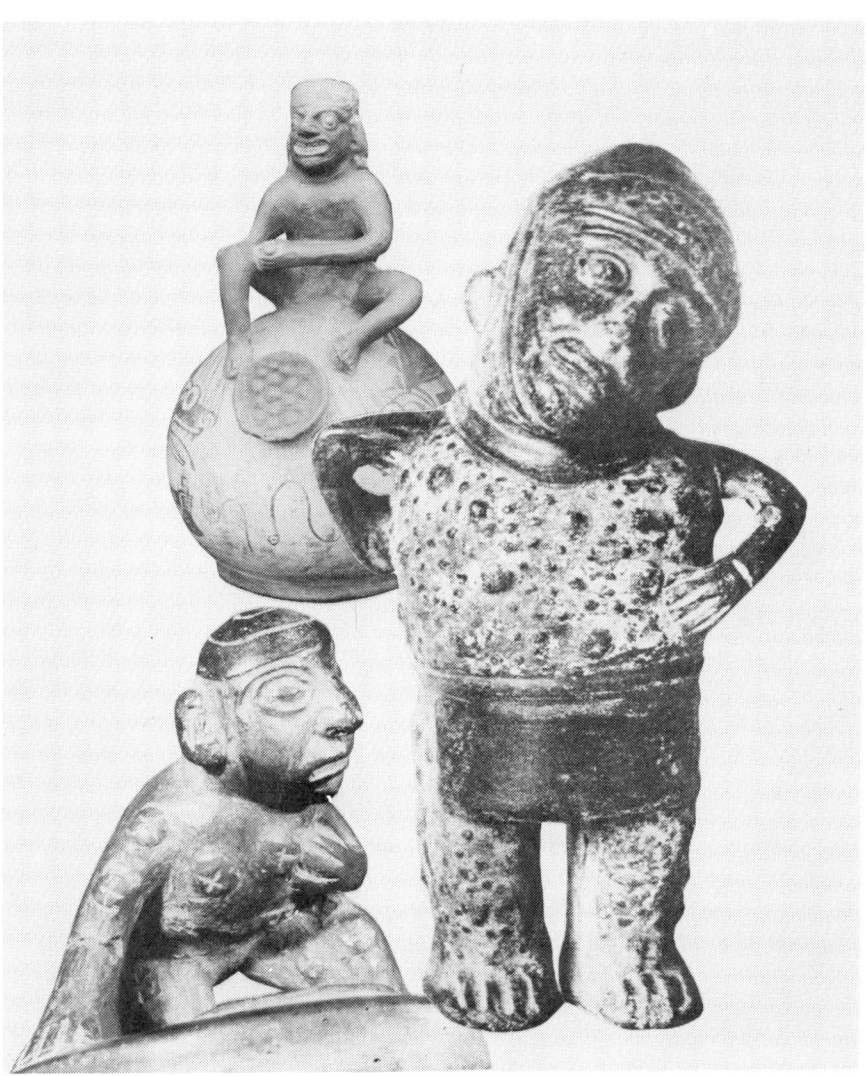

Three ceramic figures showing different skin disorders. The standing figure probably portrays a case of Peruvian verruga (see text); the man sitting on the vase is using a topical remedy on a skin rash on his thigh; the crawling man has a case of multiple common boils that have been incised in a cross-like pattern.

Because the majority of chroniclers who described the famous epidemic in Coaque, on the coast of Ecuador, used the Spanish word *verrugas*, meaning any type of warty eruption or rash, medical historians believed the Coaque disease was Peruvian verruga. Antonio de Herrera wrote during the conquest that Indians along the coast of Ecuador suffered frequently from warts on the forehead, nose, and elsewhere.[29] Spanish soldiers who camped in Coaque suffered greatly during the seven months they had to remain there; the disease sometimes killed its victims in twenty-four hours. Those who survived the first attack became covered with warts as large as hazelnuts, which bled profusely. The soldiers who did not die of the fever were unable to take care of themselves, to the point that some died of hunger and thirst. The Indians were accustomed to the disease and did not suffer such serious attacks.

Agustín de Zárate, one of the most reliable chroniclers of the period, stated that Coaque was a very unhealthy area because of the wart disease, which he described as worse than *bubas*.[30] Miguel de Estete, the soldier-writer, commented that Coaque seemed a most agreeable place were it not for its malignant atmosphere. He asserted that this disease had never been seen in the Western World.[31]

Pedro Pizarro described it in even greater detail, stating that sometimes the warts were as big as eggs, bursting and bleeding profusely; others were very small, similar to the eruptions in measles or smallpox, but they covered the body and caused it to swell up.[32]

These descriptions probably refer to what we now call Peruvian verruga, perhaps complicated by a form of acute malaria or some other explosive infectious process, and, in some cases, by food poisoning. We infer the latter from the fact that some chroniclers state that the disease occurred after an individual had eaten a certain type of fish that later proved to have been poisonous.

Today Peruvian verruga never occurs along the coast or in the jungle; it is an endemic disease found only at altitudes of between 800 and 1,500 meters. Whether its geographic distribution and intensity have changed, which is not a rare event in medical history, or whether the Coaque epidemic was produced by another disease, or a combination of diseases, such an outbreak has never recurred in either Peru or Ecuador.

MERCURY

According to several sources, the Incas discovered mercury and developed methods for mining it. It is evident, however, that they did not use mercury for medicinal purposes or in their metallurgy. On the contrary, they were aware that it was dangerous to remain in the immediate vicinity of its mineral deposits, and prohibited the exploitation of the mines. This ban was revoked by the Spaniards, who needed mercury to process gold, and who sent great numbers of slaves to the mines of Huancavelica where they soon died, victims of Spanish greed. B. Salinas y Córdova, a clergyman who wrote some years after the conquest, describes how cruelly the Indians were treated by their Spanish masters, and how they became ill from the mineral powder that destroyed their lungs.[33]

"SPONGY HYPEROSTOSIS"

Skulls with a strange bone lesion, called by Hrdlicka "symmetric osteoporosis," are found with relative frequency in some pre-Columbian cemeteries along the Peruvian coast.[34] The external surface of the skull, usually smooth and uniform, shows a thickening, a very rough surface, and a spongy protuberance distributed symmetrically on both sides. Williams studied this phenomenon in great detail and found it present among all social classes and age groups in a great many pre-Columbian coastal areas.[35] As no evidence of the condition is found in contemporary Peruvian skulls, it is difficult to identify this disorder with any known present-day disease. Weiss and H. Hamperl have made careful observations from which they concluded it was probably a disease related to anemia, perhaps malaria, which secondarily produced hypertrophy of the surface of the bone by an excessive reaction of the blood-forming organs in the bone marrow located in the spongy part of the flat bones of the skull.[36] In this sense Weiss shows the impropriety of calling this disease osteoporosis—an excessive increase in the porosity of the bone; it is a "spongy hyperostosis," an excessive development of the spongy areas of the bone.

To explain these findings on the basis of a serious reaction to malaria, or to any other contemporary disorder producing anemia, it would be necessary to find contemporary skulls showing the same lesion, which has never been done. While some types of anemia may produce similar but not identical lesions, most anemias that produce these modifications in the bone are of a hereditary type not found among Peruvians. Oscar Urteaga Ballón believes that in pre-Columbian times there may have been a hereditary disorder that produced this type of anemia, and that the disease had ceased to exist by the time the Spaniards arrived, due to the normal tendency of all degenerative diseases to disappear through the progressive interference they exert on human reproduction.*

---

* Oscar Urteaga Ballón: personal communication.

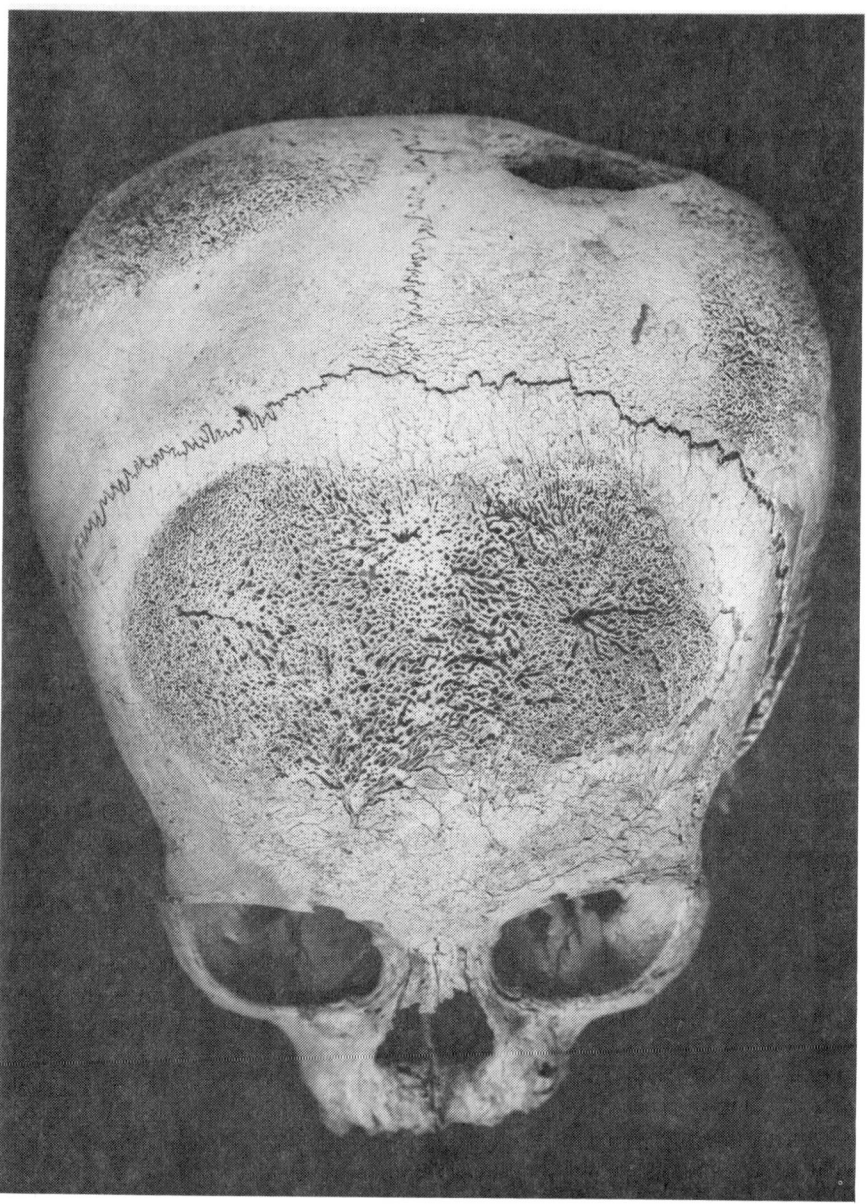

A case of so-called "spongy hyperostosis," probably the result of healed scurvy (Huaura culture).

VITAMIN C DEFICIENCY

We have postulated that the skull lesions described in this paper are very similar to those caused by scurvy, a disorder resulting from a lack of vitamin C in the diet, which was probably not infrequent among the ancient Peruvian population. Their diet was not always well balanced, and annalists often spoke of famines during the era of Incan expansion. Once the empire was well organized, despite its excellent economic and agricultural administration, it is possible that climatic and atmospheric changes may occasionally have seriously hindered the production of food. This may be inferred also from the frequency and solemnity with which Indian priests prayed to the gods to protect their harvests. Among the many Incan prayers we know of, some reveal an intense concern with the avoidance of famines.

On the other hand, although ancient writings describe the excellent diet enjoyed during normal times, it is clear that religious fasting occurred frequently and that it was sometimes abused. The most common religious fasting ritual, *sasi*, required abstinence from salt, chili, and sexual pleasures for varying periods, in some cases for as long as a year. As we know, chili—*uchu, ají, chili*—constitutes a source of vitamin C. When fasting was prolonged, therefore, as in the case of the so-called *hatun-sasi*, which required consuming only raw corn and water for several weeks or even months, the possibility of serious nutritional deficiencies becomes even more evident. We might add that in archaeological deposits in Israel the skulls of humans who were subjected to deficient nutritional conditions over long periods of time show similar characteristics to those described here.

EYE DISORDERS

Disorders of the eyes were frequent. Perhaps the best known is the disease suffered by the Incan Emperor Yahuar Huaccac. *Yahuar* means blood, and *huacca* means to cry, and the emperor is said to have cried tears of blood every time he encountered political problems. Naturally it is difficult to establish with any degree of certainty the specific type of disease he had: modern interpretations vary from a strange type of hemorrhagic conjunctivitis, to the presence of a vascular anomaly that conveniently bled every time the Incan was under political pressure. Francisco de Montesinos believes the emperor suffered from a disease that made his eyes bloodshot;[37] Salinas y Córdova maintains the emperor shed tears of blood at his birth, and that thereafter he did so whenever he made a sacrifice to the Sun God;[38] Father Cobo is of the opinion that every time the emperor had problems with his enemies he shed bloody tears.[39] All sources agree, however, that this ophthalmologic phenomenon first occurred when his father's political enemies kidnapped him. There is not a great amount of material with which to establish an exact diagnosis, however, so we will leave Yahuar Huaccac to rest in peace without offering a definite opinion.

Although the Incas did not frequently shed tears of blood, they did suffer from many eye diseases. López de Gomara observed that in one Peruvian mountain region blind or one-eyed men were often seen.[40] He wrote that it was unusual to find two people with four healthy eyes between them. Ceramic figures depict several types of blind men. P. Cieza speaks of an acute eye disease endemic in the Valley of Piura, said to be caused by the winds and sands of summer as well as by the humidity of winter.[41]

Many travellers of the sixteenth century remarked on the prevalence of *surumpi*, snow blindness, which is found throughout the world and which had evidently been appropriately identified by ancient Peruvians.

DENTAL PROBLEMS

Many dental ailments occurred with relative frequency among pre-Columbian Indians. Examples found in old graves include caries, dental abscesses, pyorrhea, and various anomalies of implantation. These have been specifically studied by several researchers, including R. Moodie,[42] A. Taiman,[43] H. García Bedoya,* and Dabbert.[44] The flattening or corrosion of the crown found in the teeth of many ancient skulls appears to be related to the habit of chewing coca with strongly alkaline and abrasive substances.

MENTAL FUNCTIONS

One problem of great interest to paleopathologists is the interpretation of skull trephining as a cultural element. The pre-Columbian Peruvians believed that mental functions were located in the cardiac region, which they called *soncco*. The word that identified the heart also designated the sources of intelligence, reason, memory, and instincts. Huamán-Poma, one of the most reliable Indian chroniclers, writes that, after her marriage, the fifth Coya, Chimbo Mama Cawa, wife of Capac Yupanqui, suffered from a disease of the heart. When she had this ailment she had attacks at least three times a day, during which she screamed outrageously, attacked people, bit and scratched, and pulled out her hair. Huamán-Poma main-

---

* H. García Bedoya: personal communication, 1956.

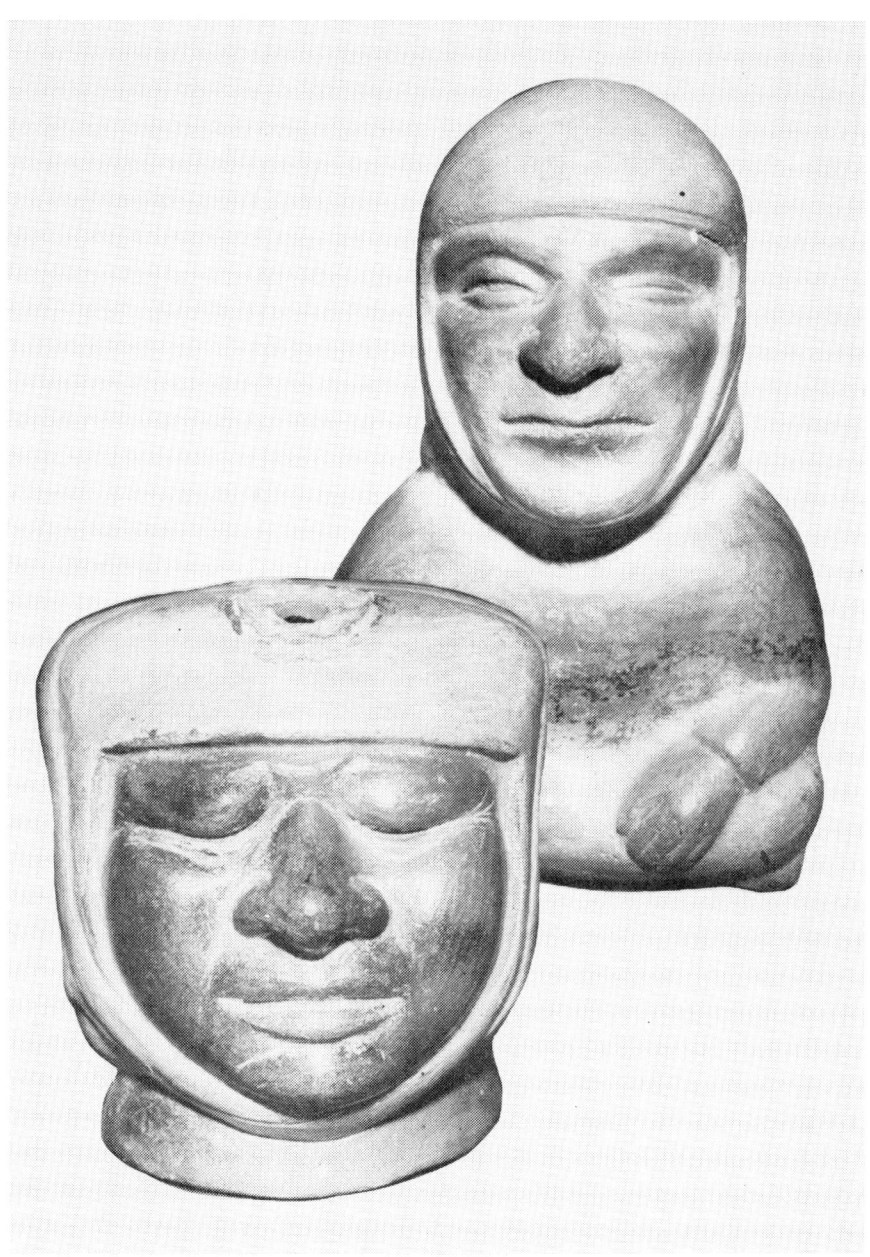

Two cases of blindness.

tains that because of this disease of the heart the Coya "became very ugly." Finally, she committed an act of canibalism on one of her children, and soon after died.[45] It is clear that Huamán-Poma was describing a mental disease even though he attributed it to the heart. Inca Garcilaso wrote that one of his uncles, a nobleman of the Inca family, told him to memorize the traditions he was being told about and "keep them in his heart," in other words, in his mind.[46]

The anecdotes points up the definite role ancient Peruvians gave the cardiac viscera with regard to spiritual functions, and the lesser role they gave the brain. To them the heart was the *sensorum comune*, as Aristotle had concluded independently, the center of all instinctive and spiritual life. Thus epilepsy was considered a cardiac disease. When considering the reason Indian surgeons trephined the skull, therefore, one should be very careful about accepting the theory that epilepsy, melancholia, and other mental disorders were "inevitable" reasons for trephining: such a deduction falls into the trap of using our present knowledge to interpret the problems of that era.

In the cultural evolution of the Incas it is difficult to pinpoint when the head assumed importance; it is even harder to estimate when the logical connection between the brain and its functions was established. It is true that most primitive peoples identify parts of the head with certain vital functions; and the most superficial observer cannot escape the importance of the eyes, ears, nose, upper respiratory passages, mouth, and vocal cords. The logical relationship of certain important functions to the head may also be established very quickly, as a trauma in this region has obvious consequences. But, paradoxically, a very long time can pass before a cultural group recognizes the logical association of the brain and its related activities. Even the most sophisticated cultures of the past struggled long and hard before discovering what now seems so obvious. They related spiritual affairs to the abdomen or to the thoracic viscera, which, after all, have a physiology that is difficult to understand.

Ancient Peruvians did not escape these rules of human knowledge. They of course assigned a primary role to the head in determining individuality, as is evident from the importance they attributed to it for individual and cultural identification—head trophies, head-dresses, tribal hats, etc.—as well as in the elaborate medical and surgical care they gave to head wounds. But it is clear that they placed mental activities in the cardiac viscera. The word *soncco* appears in almost all phrases relating to psychiatry and neurology. Neither the word *uma*, head, nor *ñutco*, brain, appears in this connection, except for such phrases that mean good memory, *ancha-umanuan hopik*, and bad memory, *mana-umayok*.

The conclusions to be drawn from these observations on linguistics must not of course be accepted dogmatically, but as guides to possible ways the thinking of pre-Columbian Peruvian philosophers might have evolved. It is true that the development of a culture is reflected in its speech patterns, but language never advances at the same pace as the historical development of knowledge. If a language specialist were to study our present manner of expressing ourselves, he would, for example, quickly discover that even in the most depurative scientific circles we call a marked psychological depression melancholia, a term that in fact means black bile. And our best poetic works—as well as those of the Incas—place the emotions in the heart: we still love, hate, and have courage because of the heart. Although the prefix "neuro" appears in the formation of many words related to the function of the nervous system, terms that relate epilepsy to the brain— cerebral dysrhythmia, centroencephalic epilepsy, cerebral crisis—were incorporated into our lexicon only very recently.

MENTAL ILLNESS

In the merger of magic and science that characterized Peruvian medicine there were undoubtedly diseases we would call psychosomatic, which may have constituted a high percentage of the disturbances treated by physicians of ancient Peru. We can acquire some knowledge of the symptomatology of these ailments from the somewhat obscure chronicles of the sixteenth century; perhaps a more accurate idea may be gained, however, by studying primitive medical practices and the interpretations of contemporary Peruvian medicine men and healers, who refuse to accept Western medical practices and continue to carry out many ancient rituals. In this regard we must give credit to a group of Peruvian psychiatrists who, working in different directions, have arrived at similar conclusions. The greater part of the information that follows was obtained from the works of H. Valdizán and A. Maldonado,[47] F. Sal y Rosas,* and C.A. Seguín;† the author's personal contribution to this field does not go beyond thorough bibliographic research.

There is, for example, a group of symptoms called *kaika*‡ that manifests itself in headaches, nausea, vomiting, general malaise, and

---

* F. Sal y Rosas: personal communication, 1962.
† C.A. Seguín: personal communication, 1971.
‡ The origin of this term is obscure. It might derive from the word *kai*, which was used to designate an invisible and omnipotent deity; it could also come from one of the local languages that are now extinct.

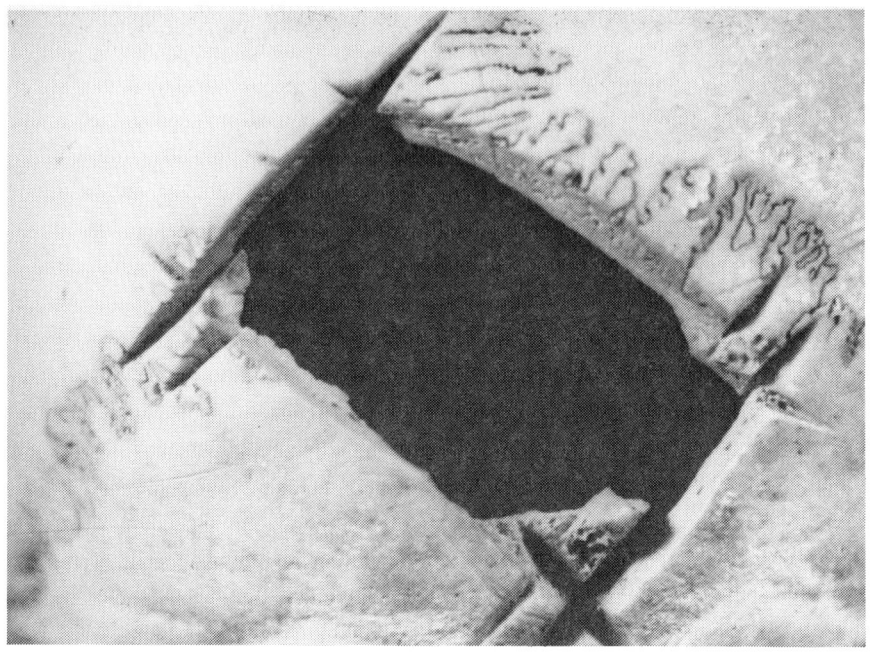
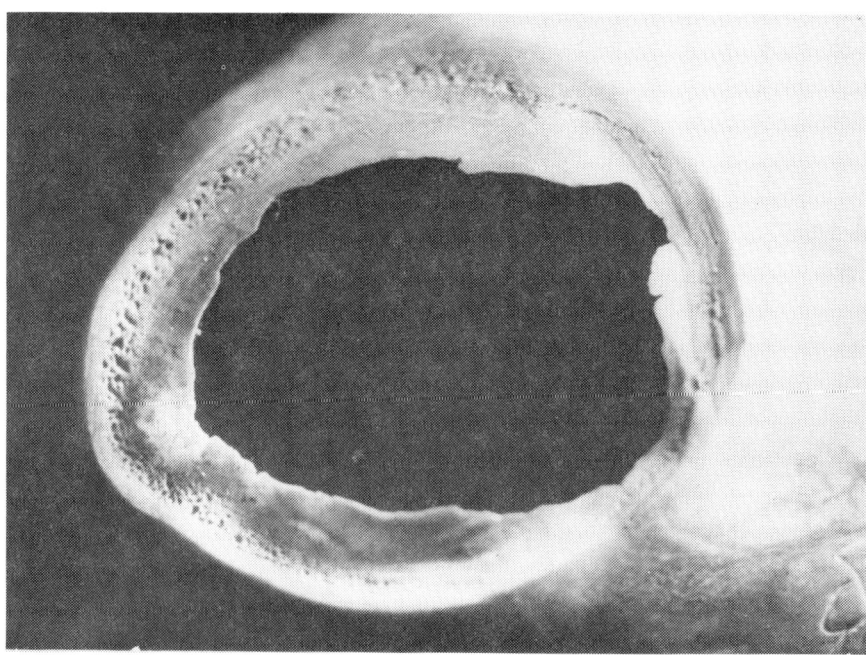

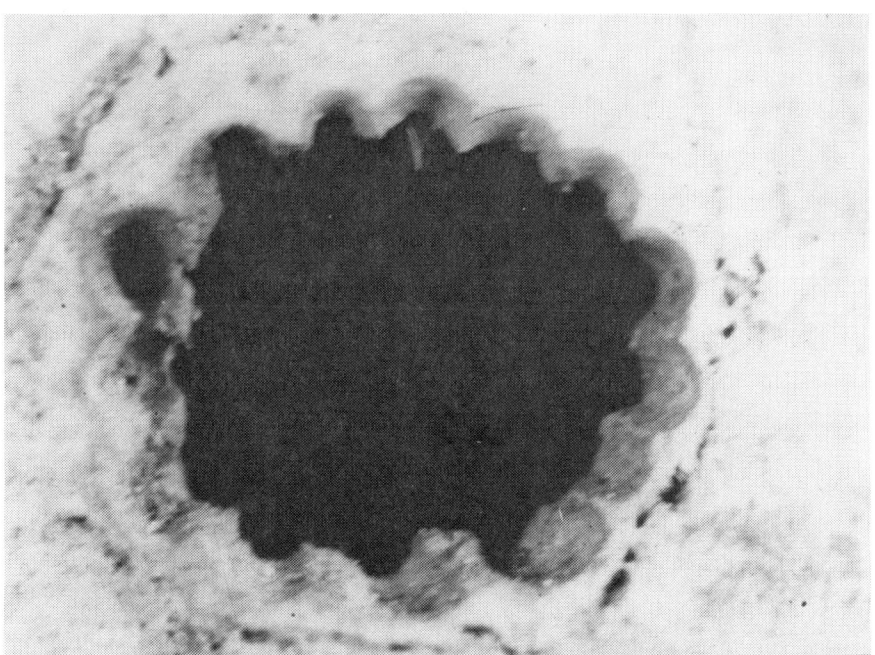

Three methods employed by pre-Columbian Peruvian surgeons to open the skull. *Opposite page top:* the square or polygonal type formed by straight bone incisions, probably performed with an obsidian knife; *bottom:* the round type produced by rasping with an abrasive stone; *above:* the multiple-trephine performed with a rotating tool.

profuse sweating. Frequently this syndrome appears after the patient has been at a very high altitude or has attended a funeral. It is an acute disorder usually followed by a prolonged illness, characterized by lack of appetite, loss of weight, mental depression, and other signs of a generalized organic imbalance. *Kaika* is generally cured through acts of magic, the one most often used being to "pay the earth"—by offering food to "mother earth."

More interesting still is the symptom called *susto*, fright, which in Quechua is called *jani*. According to contemporary Indian healers this is produced by the alienation of the soul—abandoned by the spirit, the body loses its balance and the disorder develops. The soul may be "stolen" by a mountain, a ravine, a lake, the night, a tomb, or any geographic phenomenon. The general alienation is produced by a sudden fright, but it may also occur in an insidious and slow manner. Sal y Rosas, with Western medical

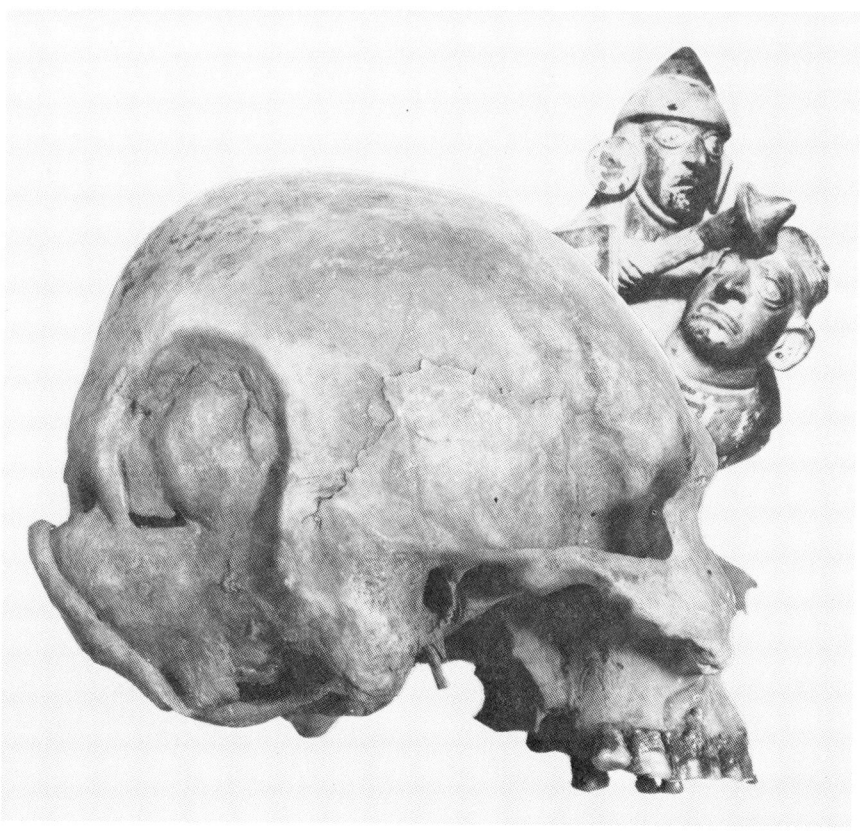

Skull showing a well-healed massive fracture of the occipital region. Survival of this patient must have entailed excellent medical care.

techniques, has studied a series of 176 cases diagnosed as *susto* and treated by contemporary native healers. He maintains that the disorder occurs at all ages, although it is very rare in mature adults. Generally the patient loses appetite, becomes pale and withered, pays very little attention to personal hygiene, and develops a great thirst. Sometimes there is moderate fever, vomiting, and diarrhea. These somatic symptoms are always accompanied by nervousness, anxiety, depression, nightmares, and generalized fear. Only in very advanced cases does the patient have to remain in bed.

The majority of patients studied by Sal y Rosas were identified by him as being victims of infectious metabolic diseases that can be identified. In such cases the psychological reactions are susceptible to treatment by native healers. In others, an organic disease that cannot be identified by modern methods has been described by Sal y Rosas as purely psychological, and it is with those cases that the healers have had greatest success. On the basis of the diagnostic requirements of the healer, Sal y Rosas has classified nine such instances as typical cases of *susto*, a group of symptoms unleashed by severe psychological trauma with the psychosomatic characteristics described. All the cases are cured dramatically by native methods that "return the soul to the body"; the majority of the methods used correspond virtually in all details to those described 400 years ago by chroniclers and missionaries in their cruel drive against the practices of "witchcraft and idolatry" by the Indians.

Mental diseases were frequently described in early chronicles and in communications sent to their superiors by Spanish priests, who were convinced that the devil had a lot to do with the appearance of mental symptoms as he tried to recover souls that had been converted to Christianity. C. de Molina, chaplain of Cuzco Hospital, wrote that once the complete and total domination of the Spaniards over the Indian race had been achieved, various types of witchcraft were practiced that caused the subdued Indians to become ill. Some danced and jumped around constantly, saying that a sacred spirit of their ancestors had entered their bodies; some had convulsions attributed to the same cause; some went into complete seclusion in their homes, blocking the doors with enormous stones; some suddenly started to weep and to mutilate their faces and hands; and some committed suicide by leaping from precipices or by drowning themselves. Such suicides happened very frequently, "until the Lord, in his Divine Mercy, illuminated these miserable people, and all who survived this fatal bewitchment realized it was the work of a demon."[48]

In these psychiatric disorders, so well described but so badly interpreted by the Spaniards of that time, we can recognize the reaction of a confused and desperate people reacting to the events of that era.

MUTUAL AID

In Incan society those injured in wars or in accidents or incapacitated by disease necessarily constituted a very serious challenge to the activities of the community, and careful planning was required to rehabilitate them as useful citizens. Garcilaso tells us that the temporary incapacity of a productive individual was resolved by the social group by means of a mutual aid system: when a person was permanently incapacitated he was given a work program within the framework of his residual capacities.[49] Chroniclers are very specific in this sense. The deaf and dumb, for example, were not considered cripples because they could do a variety of tasks. The blind, the lame, the armless, the handless, and other physical invalids were employed in a variety of occupations: weaving, seeding cotton, watching the fields, or as musicians, poets, or keepers of tradition. Thus each became a useful component of the community instead of a burden. Even their personal lives were governed by regulations: because it was difficult for a blind or lame man to marry a normal woman, the Incas decreed that the blind should marry the blind and the crippled the crippled.

MAKING WAR

As war constituted one of the principal occupations of the average citizen, and one of the most frequent causes of death or incapacity, it was necessary to learn the use of slings, darts, bludgeons, axes, *ayllos*, and other weapons that produced serious injuries. The forces of nature were also used to the utmost advantage in battles. In the intricate orography of the Andes, attacking armies were destroyed by sudden avalanches of rocks and stones unleashed by the defenders hidden in the mountains. In attacks on cities and fortresses, incendiary projectiles were hurled by slings: red-hot stones covered with cotton, which upon arriving at their destination burned and destroyed straw roofs. Prolonged sieges of entire communities frequently resulted in famine and epidemics. The survivors of these terrible ordeals displayed mutilated bodies and limbs, extensive burns, serious nutritional deficiencies, infectious diseases, and all kinds of ailments that challenged the capacities of ancient Peruvian doctors.

ATTITUDES TOWARD DISEASE

In our efforts to understand pre-Columbian Peruvian medical practice, the most difficult aspects are those that refer to the philosophy of Incan culture, because we must interpret it in terms of European Renaissance culture, which differs from our own modern Western culture. We have to make surmises about events the Incas were unable to record, and which the Spaniards could not wholly understand.

The bulk of material available to us tells of a conflict between two cultures that established contact, not through their elite of great men but through individuals who in general had little preparation for or desire to

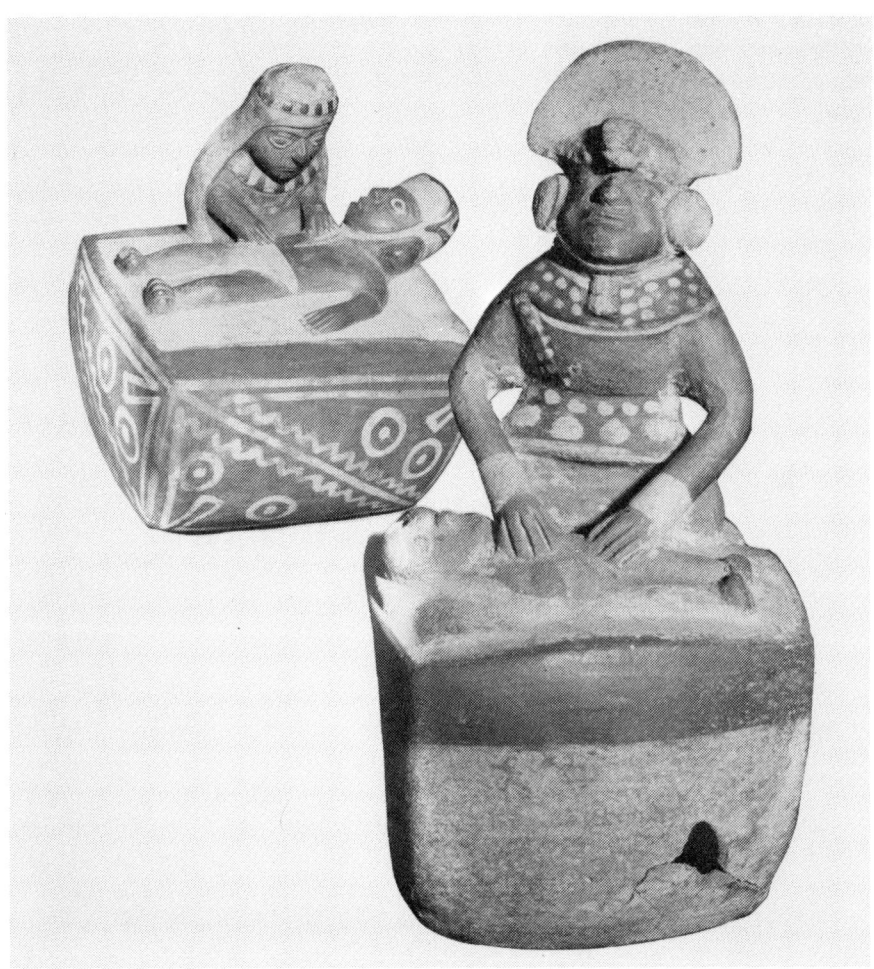

Male and female pre-Columbian Peruvian healers examining their patients.

establish a fruitful relationship. Thus many of the unknown factors that emerge step by step attract our curiosity without satisfying our thirst for accurate knowledge.

How did ancient Peruvians interpret disease? Did they perhaps consider it the product of a supernatural world, the work of the great Hanan-Pacha in some way punishing the sins of men? Or did they have empirical or scientific knowledge of the organic origins of certain diseases that could not be interpreted by the Spaniards of that time? It is true that in one way or another most of our sources insist that ancient Peruvians regarded disease as a direct result of their sins; this explanation was of course a consequence of the bizarre mixture of empiricism and magic that constituted what we now call the art of curing. But they certainly must have had many concepts not entirely compatible with that explanation. It is interesting to explore other areas of knowledge to try to decipher this complicated puzzle.

The first contradiction in their interpretation of diseases arises when we consider that the Inca was supposed to be a semi-god, a direct descendant of the Sun God, and therefore virtually infallible and free of sin. Consequently, to uphold this concept an Inca should never have become ill.

Pragmatic as they were, the Incas had a double explanation for such contradictions. Garcilaso made it very clear when he proposed that the diseases of noblemen, especially of the Incas, were considered in no way similar to those of the common man; in the case of the emperor, a disease was considered to be a message from the Sun God calling his son to rest with him in paradise. Thus when an Inca became sick and felt death approaching he simply announced, "My father is calling me to rest by his side." All sacrifice, ceremonies, and prayers for his health were thereupon cancelled.[50]

On the other hand, there are indications that the Incas had specific concepts of certain diseases that, with due respect to the supernatural world, allowed them to relate specific ailments to obvious causes. They had, for example, a distinct knowledge of the influence of the environment on health. They knew if a man from the highlands lived for any length of time in the humid valleys along the coast or in the Amazon jungle he became ill and died; on the other hand, a man from the lowlands did not easily tolerate the environment of the high, bleak plateaus or the Andean mountains. They were so conscious of these causes and effects that they based all their political and military actions on such concepts. While we do not know whether they treated such problems scientifically, their actions indicate a practical approach to human existence in different environments.

Their dual interpretation of the world gave rise to the concept of *paccarina*, which resolved the intimate connnection between the supernatural and empirical, rational deductions. Man must not leave his geographic place of origin because he is linked to it by regional gods: the mountain, lake, river, ocean, jungle, or high plateau. If he moves to another place he is committing a great sin against his god and, equally important, the rules of the empire, and he is therefore punished with a disease. Huamán-Poma has clearly established that "there were diseases from the rainbow, the fountains, the earth, and the great disease from the sacred temples."[51]

The Incas observed that certain regions were cursed with specific diseases they identified with water, plants, or the presence of a deity who to them was a jealous guardian of her territories. It was known, for example, that any foreigner who came to the sanctuary of Huamachuco, in the so-called Temple of Ataguju, contracted a disease characterized by an itching body, followed by worms eating up the flesh, and then death.

A regional disease, Peruvian verruga, caused the death of many workers when the Trans-Andean Railroad was being built during the mid-nineteenth century. While we now know that this disease was transmitted by a small mosquito indigenous to that area, only a century ago scientists attributed it to a lack of hygiene, unsanitary water, the special air of that region, and other factors, which from a practical standpoint could perfectly well have been given the name of a local deity.

Many years of observation had convinced ancient Peruvians that it was not healthy to sleep near rivers or fresh-water reservoirs in the valleys along the coast. They reached the conclusion that the mosquitoes kept them awake, and many of those who did fall asleep became ill and died. They believed that Mayo, god of the rivers, was probably punishing them for resting in his presence. Thus for centuries the Indians built their houses and communities far from the rivers, on the slopes of nearby hills where there was no water; by so doing they could not be reached by the zealous god of the water. After the Spaniards arrived the Indians were forced once again to build their communities near the rivers, where they quickly succumbed to the scourge of malaria.

They also believed that a disease could easily be produced by the direct action of a poison provided by a witch, although the origin of such toxic substances and the manner of administering them were not revealed. The only means of escape from the effects of such a disease was for the victim to appeal to another witch to counterattack the disease—a situation very similar to that of our modern iatrogenic disorders.

TRANSMISSION OF DISEASE

We do not know the extent to which ancient Peruvians were aware of the role played by some insects in the transmission of disease. All chroniclers at the time of the conquest mention the evident relationship between the unhealthiness of certain areas and the presence of great swarms of mosquitoes; but it is not known if this was deduced by the Spaniards themselves or if it was pointed out to them by the Indians.

In this regard another interesting observation has been made. In certain regions of Peru where the people were very poor and dirty, as well as in sections of better developed communities where some lived under very poor conditions, at one time the Incas decreed that these people should pay tribute in the form of small containers of lice. According to certain chroniclers this was done because whatever their economic condition all people had to acquire the habit of paying tribute to the Incas; other chroniclers maintain that the essence of the decree was to force the population to eradicate parasites and to keep themselves clean. Whatever the intention, it is interesting that 400 years later the conclusion was reached that typhus, a very common disease in ancient Peru, is in fact transmitted by lice.

Since nobody is free of sin or immune to disease, it is easy to conclude how one might be related to the other, and thus one must apply that finding or theory so that it does not upset the nucleus of the logical relationship. This was done very efficiently by ancient Peruvians, who were able to explain many aspects of pathology within the framework of the supernatural world.

For example, the infectiousness of specific diseases did not escape their observation. Their medical concept, however, was that the symptoms were probably caused by the presence of an irate deity who had invaded the home and all of its appurtenances. Consequently, they tried to free themselves of this inconvenient guest by passing it on to another person, in the belief that the best way to rid themselves of the deity was to give the disease to someone else. Father M. de Morúa states that when a man contracted a relatively serious disease, and especially when he had a high fever, he was placed by the roadside and the community prayed that the first person to come along would carry the disease away. At other times they put the patient's clothes by the roadside, in the hope that someone might steal them, and thus the disease also; this happened quite frequently. As the majority of patients thus "treated" recuperated "spontaneously," and since those who took the clothes or touched the patient in passing often contracted the disease, the logic is clear—so clear that it degenerated into a perversion.[52]

Father Cobo tells us that, on the assumption that an infuriated god wanted to take a human life, once a witch had reached the conclusion that a patient was going to die it was not unusual for the patient to kill his own son to appease the god and thus save his own life. Fortunately, this practice was frowned upon by Incan authorities and it was therefore rarely employed.[53]

After reading descriptions of the great epidemic of 1544 in Peru, we

DISEASES IN ANCIENT PERU

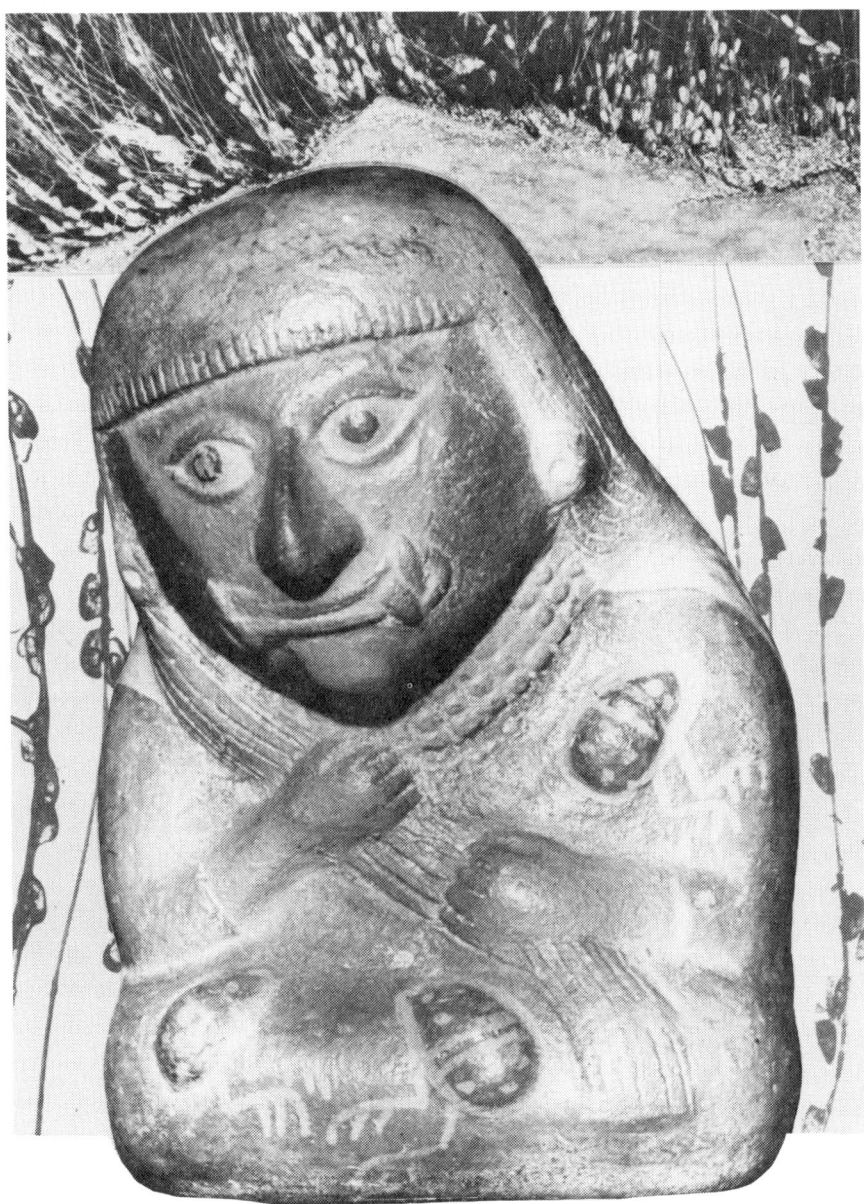

A composite photograph of a Mochica woman infested by fleas; the scalp of a Chancay mummy full of lice; and a microscopic picture of nits from the same specimen.

must conclude that Peruvians had developed the practice of protecting the individual from disease. The epidemic attacked only llamas and alpacas, and, as Garcilaso and others point out, it was highly contagious and spread rapidly, causing the deaths of two-thirds of these animals.

In a natural catastrophe of this nature, it was not the new Spanish masters but the local Indian authorities who solved the problem. There is sufficient evidence to conclude that the Indians gave orders to immediately sacrifice any animal that showed the first symptoms of the disease and to bury the carcass deep in the earth. They prohibited direct contact between the shepherds and the dead animals, and issued an edict expressly banning the consumption of their flesh. These measures, which brought the epidemic under control, are similar to procedures we would follow today under similar circumstances.

THE GOD-GERM CONCEPT

Chroniclers do not tell us how the Indians explained this method of putting an end to the epidemic. Perhaps they thought the destruction and burial of the animals appeased the gods responsible for the disease; if this were so we find ourselves with a problem of semantics. An admirer of Incan culture could suggest that in fact their concept of a god was similar to our concept of a germ.

Garcilaso mentions a type of poison used for Incan arrows. Those preparing the poison amputated the leg of a dead warrior, hung it out in the sun, and stuck arrowheads into the rotting flesh. After several days they took the arrowheads out and, without cleaning them, placed them in the shade to dry; later they assembled the arrows. This process produced a highly toxic poison for which there was no known antidote.[54]

Thus the Incans prepared a magic compound to put on their arrowheads, a magic power they cultivated on dead human flesh under the warmth of the Sun God. They even called the substance a god. We call it a germ, which grows in human protein under the agreeable warmth of the sun, and which, once cultivated, cannot be exposed to ultraviolet light because it becomes sterilized; if injected subcutaneously in man it produces an infection that is usually fatal.

But did the Incas call it a god? Some Spaniards who came to Peru— and many who remained in Spain—had no specific name for such a substance either; it was a poison, a venom. For them it was as toxic as the herbs used in witchcraft with which the Indian made magic passes over those same arrows. All Quechuan words used to designate different toxins—

many of which have disappeared—had to be translated into Spanish. But at that time it would not have been possible to translate into Spanish the Quechuan words designating such substances. Nor was there any concept in their culture—except for a very generalized knowledge of magic and witchcraft—that would allow the Spaniards to interpret what they saw on the poisonous arrows. Perhaps, then, we are faced with a linguistic rather than a biological problem—in any event a problem of comparative ethnology.

DIAGNOSIS

It is curious to note that Garcilaso, the greatest encomiast of Incan culture, when evaluating the medical concepts of ancient Peruvian healers, commented with great sorrow that Incan physicians "could not recognize the body fluids by looking at urine."[55] He wrote this at a time when European physicians were resolving their most difficult problems by taking a bottle of the patient's urine and looking at it against the light with solemn academic countenances. This method, called uroscopy, was at that time believed by experts to be an accurate and scientific way to make a diagnosis. For Garcilaso, who by then had been exposed to the Western world, Indian doctors were not aware of this method and therefore, sad to state, they were "backward."

They were indeed backward. To decide how to treat a patient Incan physicians resorted to using guinea pigs, spiders, coca leaves, and magic rituals. Then, almost in passing, they took the patient's pulse, looked at his tongue, felt the temperature of his skin, palpated his stomach, and sat and listened for a long while to what the patient had to say. But they did not know how to look at urine.

Father Cobo fell into the same trap, not in spite of but because of his own knowledge of Renaissance medicine. In his long dissertation on Peruvian medicine he criticizes the diagnostic capacity of the Indians on the basis of their lack of medical terminology;[56] despite the fact that they were older men with long experience with the sick, they did not know how to classify diseases or give them their proper names. Cobo should have realized that the concept and classification of diseases in the Incan culture were so different from those of Renaissance Europe that there was no point in making comparisons or direct translations because both sides became confused when they tried to understand each other in languages that were totally different, as were their cultures.

It would be interesting to learn what concepts ancient Peruvians held on pathogenisis—the way in which a certain disease creates the symptoms that characterize it. Following a universal pattern, they explained the production of symptoms either by the penetration of an extraneous agent into the patient—call it a poison, an herb, a magic spirit, a parasite, or a germ—or by the separation of any of a person's normal components. Both produce an imbalance that is incompatible with health. Regarding primitive medical thinking, H.E. Sigerist, the noted American medical historian, states that, "Man becomes ill because there is something in his body that is not his, or because something has been taken away from his body which is necessary for him to live."[57]

Basically, then, the culture of the ancient Peruvians had reached a firm basis that would enable them to understand the concept of disease, and they had a well-organized framework in which they could place the results of their observations. Unfortunately, much of the knowledge their wise men accumulated during centuries of work has been lost to our civilization in the painful intercultural whirlwind.

NOTES

1. A. Hrdlicka, *Anthropological Work in Peru in 1913, with Notes on the Pathology of Ancient Peruvians* (Washington: n.p., 1914).
2. R. Moodie, "Studies in Paleopathology. XVIII. Tumors of the Head among Pre-Columbian Peruvians," *Annals of Medical History* 8 (1926):397.
3. _____, "Studies in Paleopathology. XXI. Injuries to the Head among the Pre-Columbian Peruvians," *Annals of Medical History* 9 (1927):227.
4. _____, "Studies in Paleopathology. XXIII. Surgery in Pre-Columbian Peru," *Annals of Medical History* 11 (1929):690.
5. H.U. Williams, "Human Paleopathology," *Archives of Pathology* 7 (1929): 839.
6. J.C. Tello, *La Antigüedad de la Sífilis en el Peru* (Lima: n.p., 1909).
7. P. Weiss, "Restos Humanos de Cerro Colorado," *Revista Museo Nacional de Lima* 1 (1932): 3.
8. _____, "Origen Americano de las Treponemiasis: Sífilis y Mal de Pinto," *Revista Ginecología y Obstetricia* 2 (1956): 41.
9. _____, "Osteología Cultural," *Annals de la Facultad de Medicina de Lima* 41 (1958):505.
10. J.B. Lastres et al., *Representaciones Patológicas en la Cerámica Peruana* (Lima: n.p., 1943).
11. J.B. Lastres, *La Medicina Incaica* (Lima: n.p., 1951).
12. O. Dabbert, "Contribucíon a la Paleopatología Pre-Columbina," Doctoral thesis, Universidad de Lima Facultad de Medicina, 1957.
13. Hrdlicka, *Pathology of Peruvians* (See note 1).
14. Fray Antonio de la Calancha, *Crónica Moralizada de la Orden de San Agustín en el Perú* (Barcelona: n.p. 1638).
15. J.C. Tello, *La Antigüedad de la sífilis en el Perú* (Lima: n.p., 1909).
16. Antonio Herrera, *História General de los Hechos de los Castellanos en las Islas y Tierra Firme del Mar Océano* (1604?; Buenos Aires: n.p. 1945).
17. Francisco López de Gomara, *História General de las Indias* (1554; Madrid: n.p., 1932).
18. J.C. Tello and H. Williams, "An Ancient Syphilitic Skull from Paracas in Peru," *Annals of Medical History* 12 (1930):515.

19. A.V. Kidder and E. Hooton, as cited in H.U. Williams, "The American Origin of Syphilis," *Archives of Dermatology and Syphilis* 16 (1927): 683.
20. G.F. Eaton, "The Collection of Osteological Material from Maccu-Picchu," *Memoirs of the Connecticut Academy of Arts and Sciences* (1916).
21. G. McCurdy, "Human Skeletal Remains from the Highlands of Peru," *American Journal of Physical Anthropology* (1923).
22. P. Weiss, "Probable Etiología Palúdica de la Espongiohiperostosis que se Encuentra en los Cráneos de lo Antiguos Peruanos," *Annals de la Facultad de Medicina de Lima* 39 (1956):1027.
23. Pedro Pizarro, *Descubrimiento y Conquista del Perú* (XVI century; Lima: n.p., 1927).
24. Fernando de Santillan, *Relación del Origen, Descendencia, Política, y Gobierno de los Incas. Tres Relaciónnes de Antigüedades Peruanas* (1572; Buenos Aires: n.p. 1950).
25. Fray Rodrigo Loayza, *Memorial de las Cosas del Perú Tocantes a los Indios* (1586) (Collection of unedited documents on the history of Spain, volume 44, Madrid, 1889).
26. F. Huamán-Poma de Ayala, *Nueva Crónica y Buen Gobierono* (1580-1620; Paris: n.p., 1936).
27. Moodie, "Tumors" (See note 2).
28. J.E. García Frías, "La Tuberculosis de los Antiguos Peruanos," Paper presented at the 27th International Congress of the Americas (Lima: n.p. 1942).
29. Herrera, *História General* (See note 16).
30. Agustín de Zárate, *História del Descubrimiento y Conquista del Perú* (Seville: n.p., 1577).
31. Miguel de Estete, *Noticia del Perú. Bibliografica de Cultura Peruana* (Lima: Horacio Urteaga, 1938).
32. Pizarro, *Conquista del Perú* (See note 23).
33. Buenaventura Salinas y Córdova, *Memorial de las Histórias del Nuevo Mundo. Perú.* (Lima: Gerónimo de Contreras, 1630).
34. Hrdlicka, *Pathology of Peruvians* (See note 1).
35. Williams, *Human Paleopathology* (See note 5).
36. H. Hamperl and P. Weiss, "Uber die Spongiose Hyperostose an Schadeln aus Alt Perú," *Virchows. Bd.* 327 (1955): 629.
37. F. de Montesinos, *Memorias Antiguas Históriales y Políticas del Perú* (1650?; Lima: n.p. 1930).
38. Salinas y Córdova, *Histórias del Nuevo Mundo* (See note 33).
39. Fray P. Bernabé Cobo, *História del Nuevo Mundo* (1653; Seville: n.p., 1892).
40. Gomara, *História General* (See note 17).
41. P. Cieza de Leon, *Crónica General del Perú* (1586; Madrid: n.p., 1853).
42. R. Moodie, "Studies in Paleopathology. IV. The Diseases of the Ancient Peruvians and Some Account of Their Surgical Practices," *Surgical Clinics of Chicago* (1920).
43. A. Taiman, *Anomalías Dentarias en los Antiguos Peruanos* (Lima: n.p., 1949).
44. Dabbert, "Paleopatología pre-Colombiana" (See note 12).
45. Huamán-Poma, *Nueva Crónica* (See note 26).
46. Inca Garcilaso de la Vega, *Comentarios reales de los Incas* (1609; Buenos Aires: n.p. 1943).
47. H. Valdizán and A. Maldonado, *La Medicina Popular Peruana* (Lima: n.p. 1922).
48. Cristóbal de Molina, *Relación de las Fábulas y Ritos de los Incas* (1573-75; Lima: n.p., 1916).
49. Garcilaso, *Comentarios reales* (See note 46).
50. Ibid.
51. Huamán-Poma, *Nueva Crónica* (See note 26).
52. Fray Martín de Morúa, *História del Origen y Genealogía real de los Reyes Incas del Perú* (XII century; Madrid: n.p. 1946).
53. Cobo, *Nuevo Mundo* (See note 39).
54. Garcilaso, *Comentarios reales* (See note 46).
55. Ibid.
56. Cobo, *Nuevo Mundo* (See note 39).
57. H.E. Sigerist, *A History of Medicine* (New York: n.p. 1951).

NUTRITION AND FEEDING PRACTICES OF THE MAYA IN CENTRAL AMERICA

Carlos Tejada

Dietary habits are a reflection of man's need to feed himself, and are conditioned by the characteristic culture of his society. Nutrition as a cultural complex has become so rooted within each society that it may be identified by a series of behavioral standards related to ritual practices, beliefs, taboos, traditions, and in general to an entire folklore that rotates around food and feeding practices. Which culture does not acknowledge and praise its native dishes!

Numerous factors influence the characteristics of the food and feeding habits of different societies. Among those deserving special attention are: the physical environment; the biological behavior of plants and animals; the human resources; and the technology. These will, on the one hand, delimit for us the availability of food, measured in terms of productivity and exchange, and, on the other, the size of the population, its beliefs, taboos, education, and, in general, feeding habits that define for us the demand for certain kinds of food and ways of preparing it according to the tastes of each culture. In summary, the availability of and the demand for certain kinds of food allow us to delineate the characteristics of the feeding habits of any society.

The history of a culture reveals the habits and techniques of planting, gathering, distribution, and preparation of food. It also describes for us the prestige and function of certain aliments and their relation to a great many religious, public, or family activities. Mystical beliefs within each culture are also associated with food, which explains such practices as "food for the gods" and other such offerings, as well as the prohibited kinds of food, and the fast days when food may not be eaten.

It is worth pointing out that there is a marked connection between certain cultural traits and nutrition, for example, food and health, social class, family, work, religious life, social change, folklore, social exchange, and politics. In practically every activity of human life there is a trait that is related to food. Finally, feeding habits have become so rooted in all cultures that sometimes any change therein causes severe modifications in the structure and function of a society.

This paper represents the results of research on the nutrition of inhabitants of Central America and, particularly, of the Maya.

FOOD: CORN

The Divine Manifestation of Corn and the Formation of Man

The diet of the Central American Indian, and of the great pre-Columbian cultures in general, centered around corn, which was and still is for our Indians what wheat is for the European, and rice is for the Asian.

The Indians attached the highest value to corn, and proof of this is the fact that it ceased to be merely a simple nourishment and became the creative element of man. According to the *Popol Vuh*,[1] the book that is in fact the Maya-Quiché bible, after the earth had been formed Tepeu and Gucumatz, the progenitors, "held a council in the dark of night.... and they found and discovered what should go into the flesh of man." Finally, in Paxil and Cayalá, the progenitors discovered a

> beautiful Earth, full of delights, abundant in yellow ears of corn and white ears of corn and abundant too in *pataxte* and cocoa and in innumerable *zapotes* (sapota fruits), *anonas* (custard apples), *jocotes* (corn), *matasanos*, and honey. By grinding the yellow ears of corn and the white ears of corn, Ixmucané made nine beverages, and from this nourishment came strength and stoutness, and with it they created the musculature and the vigor of man.... Only corn dough went into the flesh of our first forefathers, the four men who were created (Balam-Quitzé, Balam-Acab, Mahucutah, and Iqui-Balam).

To the Indian, the entire history of the creation of man thus begins with corn, as the *Popul Vuh* reveals when describing the supernatural role it was given within our culture.

Corn was deified by the Maya. In the *Codex Dresdensis* it is identified in the Mayan pantheon as a young divinity with an ear of corn or a bird as a head ornament. In addition, he wore a bag of *copal* hanging from his neck.

In the codices this deity is always accompanied by the sign *Kan*, the symbol of corn in the codices and the day of which this deity was the patron.²

In Mayan mythology this god had many hostile, as well as friendly, gods to whom his destiny was closely linked—the gods of the wind, of the rain, of hunger, and of death. His original name is unknown, but in the postclassic period with its Tolteca influence he is confused with an agricultural deity who was known by the name of Yum Kax, or lord of the forests. Like the mighty Chac and Itzamná, he was a good god to whom the Maya offered their sacrifices in exchange for prosperity and abundant crops.

The Orign of Corn

While all archaeologists accept the fact that corn is a native American product, there is no unanimous opinion as to the exact place on the continent where it was grown domestically for the first time.

Some researchers such as P.C. Mangelsdorf and J.W. Cameron believe corn originated in the Peruvian Andes.³ They argue that in Peru a variety of species of corn exists that is comparatively greater than that to be found in the other American countries.

Other researchers believe corn developed in Central America, specifically in the west on the central plateau of Guatemala. This is the only region where *teocinte* and *tripsacum* grow, plants that philogenetically are more primitive than corn itself and from which it could have descended. In Guatemala there are two varieties of *teocinte*, one perennial and the other annual, and several species of *tripsacum*. These are the only two plants that can be crossed with corn, a fact that permits S.G. Morley to reach the conclusion that "the highlands of northern Middle America have a better claim to having been the region where Indian corn originated than have the highlands of Peru."⁴

Going somewhat deeper into this, in Guatemala there are varieties of corn that modern biologists have been able to classify. The historian Fray Francisco Ximénez says in this regard:

> And truthfully, wheat is native to those lands from which their usual bread is made. And just as God put many different strains in wheat—whitish, gold and others—he also put them in corn. There are others: white, red, black, and purple, and painted, and among them is one called *zacpor*, which puffs up very much; it is used to make crullers and other foods for gifts. There is another very small corn, which if roasted bursts and opens in such a way that it puffs up very much; this corn roasted in this way is called *bonbon* and it is a tasty

thing when hot. Another type of corn is small; it produces a small ear of corn and is planted like wheat, whereas all the others are planted in clusters of three and four grains together. There is another type that does not produce an ear like the others . . . its grains are in the tassel, like wheat.[5]

In summary, Morley mentions three theories to explain the origin of corn:

> 1) development from *teocinte* by the orthodox biological methods of variation, mutation, and selection; (2) hybridization of *teocinte* and some unknown member of the grass family; and (3) development from some extinct, or at least as yet unknown, pre-maize plant.[6]

The Corn Growing System—The Corn Field

The system of growing corn has not changed substantially during the last 3,000 years, that is, since the preclassic era of the culture of Central America. The only change has been in the use of different agricultural tools, from the *xul* (sowing stick)* and *bat* (stone hatchet) to the use of the hoe, the axe, and the *machete*, all modern steel tools that perform the same tasks, although more efficiently.

On the high plateaus of Guatemala and on the plains of Petén and Yucatán, corn was planted in plots, usually on forest land where humus was abundant. The bushes, lianas, and small trees were usually felled by a *bat*; the big trees died out after cross-sections had been cut into the trunks. The felled scrubs were burned in March, April, and May, before the rains, when the dead leaves were completely dry. This burning, which is still practiced, is called *roza* and is done on a dry, sunny, and very windy day.

This operation was accompanied by an invocation to the gods, and apparently the priests chose the favorable days very carefully. In Copán the *Stelas* 10 and 12, which are built on two opposite hills surrounding the valley six-and-one-half kilometers apart, served as lookouts to observe the sunset in such a way that the sun sets directly behind *Stela* 10 on 12 April, which coincides precisely with the time the burnings are begun in the entire region.[7]

The priests also utilized their codices to choose the days for the burning, as may be seen in the *Codex Peresianus*, which contains numerous *tonalmatls* with divine figures, the characteristic day, and number signs of

---

* A long rod with a point hardened by fire. The growing of corn is covered in several stages by various colonial annalists, as well as by modern travelers and researchers.

this ritual computation. Prior to sowing in the month of May when the rains began, a light cleaning was made followed by the ritual ceremony. Holes were made in the ground with the planting stick, at a predetermined distance apart, and the grains of corn were placed in each one. Thereafter the holes were closed with the foot or with the planting stick.

The next stage was the weeding of the field. Weeds were pulled out by the root, unlike the present procedure whereby cutting is done with a *machete* in order to prevent competition from the weeds.[8] After the grain ripened the canes were bent in order to prevent rain from penetrating the ears of the corn and to prevent birds from eating the grains. Finally, beginning in December the harvest began and the ears and grains were stored in barns.

This ancient system of sowing remains unchanged, defying time as a live technique, a mixture of tradition and habit, religion and source of life. Fray Diego de Landa, the Yucatecan chronicler of the period immediately after the conquest, describes the cultivation of corn as follows:

> There are the tillers and those who go to pick the corn and the other seeds, which they keep in very pretty silos and barns to be sold in due time. Their mules and oxens are the people. They are wont to plant for each married man and his wife a measure of 400 feet, which they called *hum uinic*, measured with a rod of twenty feet, twenty in width, and twenty in length. The Indians have the good habit of helping one another in their work. At the time of their seed beds, those who have no families of their own to help them join in groups of twenty, more or less, and . . . do the task and do not stop until everything is done. The land, as of now, is common land and thus whoever occupies it first owns it. They sow in many parts so that in case one fails the other will supply. For tilling the land all they do is pick up the rubbish and burn it to sow thereafter. From the middle of January until April they till, and then with a pointed stick they make a hole in the earth and place in it five or six grains, which they cover with the same stick. And when it rains it is frightful how it grows.[9]

The yield of a cornfield decreased with time, and at the end of a few years, depending on the type of soil and other factors, its production no longer compensated for the effort put into it, at which time the field was abandoned. The Maya were then forced to look for other virgin land in the neighborhood for their cornfields. As long as people could count on this virgin land covered with underbrush the fate of the community was assured. When only artificial man-made savannahs remained they had to migrate. This is one of the hypotheses put forth to explain the abandonment of Tikal.[10]

Consumption of Corn

Corn was the basis of the diet of all the inhabitants of Central America. Ximénez expresses himself as follows in this regard: "Corn is the general nourishment of all those living in this America, not only of men but of animals and birds. I think there is no one who does not eat corn."[11]

The preparation of corn as a food varied from place to place: the Maya of Yucatán prepared it in the form of *pozole* (porridge), *atole* (gruel), and *tamal*,[12] the recipes for which are given by Landa in his book *Relacíon de las Cosas de Yucatán (Report of Yucatán Affairs)*, in which he writes:

> The main nourishment comes from corn, from which they make various dishes and beverages.... Indian women put the corn to soak in lime and water at night and by the next morning it is soft and half cooked and the skin and the stalk can be removed; they grind it on stones, and that which is half ground they make into big balls for the workers and travelers by land and sea,....it lasts a few months just by souring; from the rest they take a pellet and dissolve it in containers made from the skin of a fruit.... They drink that substance and eat the rest and it is tasty and of great sustenance. From the finely ground part they obtain milk and curdle it by the fire and make a sort of porridge for the morning that they drink hot; they pour water into what is left over from the morning to drink during the day because they do not drink pure water. They also roast the corn, grind it, and dissolve it in water; it is a very refreshing beverage when some India pepper and cocoa are added.[13]

It seems that the ancient Maya did not eat corn in the form of *tortillas*, which apparently were imported at a later date. For their preparation, however, the same dough referred to by Landa was used, as well as the lime and water in which to soak the grain and then cook it.

Tomas Gage, who traveled through Guatemala in 1625, describes the preparation of *tortillas* consumed by the Indians as follows:

> Their regular diet consists of *tortillas*, round patties made of corn dough that are eaten hot as they come out of a baking pan where they cook quickly.... they are eaten either plain or with chili and salt, or soaked in salt water and some crushed chili. [He describes two other ways of consuming corn: as *elote* (on the cob)] .... When the corn is still green and tender they cook the ears with the tassel and the leaves that cover it and eat it with a little bit of salt. I have eaten them many times and have found them as delicious and nutritious as our green peas, but they make the blood increase [or as *atole* (gruel)] When the corn is still green they make a sort of gruel by boiling it with milk, which they extract by crushing it. The Indians never lack for gruel, as poor as they may be, and consider themselves quite satisfied when they have enough.[14]

Cornbread is much more recent, the result of Spanish technology introduced during the colonial period. Landa tells us that "they never succeeded in making flour that can be kneaded like wheat flour; if it is made like wheat bread it is not worth eating."[15]

FOOD: BEANS

Varieties of Beans

Beans were the next most popular grain with the Maya; together with corn they formed their basic diet and covered to a great extent the caloric and protein requirements of the population. It is probable, however, that the consumption ratio of corn and beans was not satisfactory, if we accept the fact that for the present adult Guatemalan Indian the average daily consumption of corn is 423 grams, and that of beans, 58 grams. Experimental studies in animals have revealed that the optimum corn:beans ratio should be 2:6.[16] The protein deficiency in this diet was balanced with other proteins, probably of animal origin.

The variety of beans that existed in this region are described by Ximénez, who tells us that

> of these, the Divine Providence has given so many different kinds that it is a great wonder . . . . In addition to those already known in Europe called string beans, or the kidney beans of the Indies, there are many varieties of white, black, and red. Among these the one that takes first place is a kind of little kidney bean, the color of a lentil, which grows in a hot climate and reproduces in such abundance that from four grains that are sowed, four *almudes* [about three liters] may be picked. If cooked like lentils there is no difference whatsoever.
>
> There are others that are brown and white, which entwine in the corn plants and are extremely abundant . . . . [others are] very big, larger than lima beans, which grow in mountainous places; I have seen more than six varieties of these; all of them entwine and are very abundant. There are little round ones in the mountains which are all colors and which also entwine very much. There are other very small ones, like lentils, which are brownish, entwine very much, and are plentiful.[17]

Two varieties of beans are certainly indigenous to Central America: the small black bean and the red bean, the former being the favorite of most Maya and their descendants. Others, particularly the white beans, are of Spanish origin and were brought to America shortly after its discovery, as were lima beans, chick peas, and lentils.

The Growing of Beans

The beans were either planted in the same holes as the corn, so they would climb up the corn plant (corn beans), or planted separately (earth beans or creeper). The same techniques are still used. In his *Recordación Florida,* Fuentes y Guzmán writes:

> This prodigal as well as indefatigable valley yields a great number of beans of many tasty varieties, the most common and abundant being the black ones, which they call *taletes* (which corresponds in Spanish to *frisol de tierra* [earth beans] from *tali* for "earth" and *et* for "any kind of beans") because they spread on the earth in the same manner as the cucumber. There are other completely white beans, some red like coral, and bigger ones that are pitch black, which they call *vejuquillos* (small rattan), because they climb and embrace the neighboring plants.[18]

The Consumption of Beans

Beans were prepared by the Indians in different ways, some of which are similar to those used today. Usually they cooked them with chili:

> ... they keep them dry for the whole year and then they cook them with chili, with which they feel quite satisfied. They also prepare them ... by cooking the beans for a short while and mixing them with a corn dough, like we do in England with the currants in our cakes, and then they cook them together and eat them while they are still hot, or else keep them cold. But they always eat [everything] ... either with green chili, or soaked in salt water in which there is some crushed chili.[19]

Finally, as pointed out by Ximénez, "Of these and of many other varieties I have seen, they also eat them green in their pods, and make many kinds of dishes out of them."[20]

FOOD OF ANIMAL ORIGIN

Domestic Animals

In pre-Columbian American there were no large domesticated quadrupeds such as those that were a decisive factor in the development of the civilizations of the old continent. Llamas and vicuñas existed in the South American Andes and they were used by the Peruvian Indians for transportation. On the plains of North America there were buffaloes, which the Indians hunted for a twofold purpose: to use their hides for clothing and shelter and their meat for food. The buffalo was never domesticated, however. In Central America no four-legged animals were domesticated, either for use for transportation or as food. For this reason transportation was provided exclusively by slaves.

The cannibalistic practices of the Indians in various regions of the continent may be attributed to the lack of domestic animals for human consumption. As the Jesuit, Father Bernabé Cobo, wrote around the middle of the seventeenth century:

> Where this fierce habit was most accepted was where few animals could be found with whose meat the men could nourish themselves, such as on the islands of Barlovento and many other places; in regions where there were wild as well as tame animals, such as in the entire empire of the Inca kings and in some other provinces, this practice of eating human flesh did not exist.[21]

In Central America the situation was quite similar to that of the Inca empire. Although human sacrifices were frequently made, especially in the Toltec and Aztec cultures, as well as among the Maya of the postclassic period who had been in contact with and influenced by the Toltecs, they were for ritual purposes to please or ask favors of supernatural beings, and were not true man-eating practices to satisfy their appetites. There is some doubt, however, that the Aztec emperors ate human flesh habitually.[22]

In the Mayan area, particularly, hunting and fishing were very popular, and dogs and turkeys were domesticated. The dogs were small, had no coats, and did not bark. After castrating the male it was fattened with corn and utilized as food or as an offering to the gods. Dogs were used for hunting and, as Landa writes, "They do not know how to bark nor to do wrong to men, but for hunting, yes, because they make the quails and other birds rise, and they pursue the deer; some are great retrievers."[23]

Dog flesh was eaten during festivities or in times of famine. But by the beginning of the eighteenth century these dogs no longer existed, as observed by Ximénez:

> Formerly there were in these lands some small animals like dogs, the name our Spaniards gave them; they were raised by the Indians, domesticated, and did not bark. It is evident that they are a different species from our dogs. They were very good to eat and in those early days this species of dogs filled a great need as people very often died from hunger, as Bernal Díaz del Castillo points out many times. These dogs are completely extinct today and are not to be found anywhere in this kingdom of Guatemala or in what I have seen of the New Spain.[24]

In the Maya codices some figures representing deities are accompanied by these dogs; the god of lightning is also represented in the codices in the shape of a dog.[25]

The wild turkey (*Meleagris gallo pavo*) of Central America was domesticated by the Indians and used as a source of food and as an offering to the gods in sacred sacrifices; in the latter case it always had to be a wild turkey.[26] The turkey as a source of food is one of the contributions of Central America to the Western world.

Game Animals

It is important to emphasize the fact that the scarcity of domestic animals in Central America was compensated for by the great variety and abundance of game: mammals, reptiles, birds, and fish. Hunting was therefore very popular among the Maya of Yucatán. In the words of Landa, their first historian:

> There are so many deer it is marvelous, and they are small and the meat is good to eat. There are innumerable rabbits, very much like ours, except the snout, which is like that of a lamb; they are big and good to eat.[27]

They also hunted the armadillo, a fact apparently unknown to the Spaniards as Landa does not give it a specific name but simply describes it as

> a newly born sucking pig . . . it is a great rooter, covered completely by pretty shells which seem like an armor of hair, with only the little ears and the feet and hands sticking out . . . it is very good to eat and tender.[28]

Finally, there was another animal unknown in Spain, identified as *tacuatzin*.

> They are like little dogs; their heads are the shape of a pig's and they have long tails; they are the color of smoke and marvelously slow; so much so that many times they are caught by the tail. The females give birth to fourteen or eighteen little ones and God provided the mothers with a strange pouch on the belly wherein they are protected.[29]

Edible birds were also very profuse in the Yucatán and the Indians hunted them for food. In this respect Landa tells us:

> There are many field birds that are all good to eat, and three kinds of pretty little pigeons. Some birds are very simlar to the partridges of Spain, except that they have very long legs and are not good to eat. They are, however,

marvelously domesticated . . . . There are many quails, a little bigger than ours, that are exquisite to eat. The brownish and painted pheasants are of a reasonable size but not as good to eat as the ones of Italy.[30]

Fishing is not left out. Again, in the words of Landa, in Yucatán a great variety of

fish exist, and there are very excellent and very fat *lisas* (river fish); trout that are delicious to eat (in the native tongue they are called *uzcay*); very good haddock; sardines, sole, sawfish, sea horses, and innumerable varieties of other small fish; there are very good octopuses along the coast of Campeche, three or four kinds of very good and healthful spotted dogfish.[31]

The Maya of Yucatán also hunted the manatee, which was abundant along the coasts and in the estuaries:

There are many manatee on the coast between Campeche and La Desconocida which are excellent for cooking to eat. They are so big that one gets more meat from them than from a big calf, with lots of fat. The meat is good, especially when fresh; with mustard, it is almost like beef. The Indians kill them with harpoons.[32]

The iguana was a precious species of game, valued by the Indians as well as by the first conquistadores, especially in times of fasting:

There are many iguanas, which resemble the lizards of Spain in size and color, although they are not so green; they lay eggs in large amounts and are always found close to the water. The Spaniards eat them in times of fasting and find them a very healthful food. The Indians hunt them with ropes, high up on trees, and it is unbelievable how long they can go hungry; they remain alive after having been caught for twenty or thirty days without eating a bite and without getting thin. I have heard that if their bellies are rubbed with sand they get very fat. The dung of the iguana cures films on the eyes, if put fresh on them."[33]

The Indians also had other edible reptiles such as turtles, which were

marvelously big ones that are good to eat. They lay 150 to 200 eggs as big as hens. They make a large hole in the sand and cover it with the sand, and there the little turtles come out. There are other kinds of turtles that live on the ground and in the lakes.

Sometimes I saw a fish along the coast the size of a small turtle, covered on top by a delicate round shell, beautifully shaped and very bright green; its tail is also made of shell, very thin and long, like the distance from the end of the extended thumb to the end of the extended forefinger; underneath it has many feet. This fish is full of tiny eggs which the Indians eat; in their native tongue they call it *mex*.[34]

Like the Maya of Yucatán, those of the Guatemalan high plateau spent much time hunting and fishing. Ximénez, in addition to giving detailed descriptions of Guatemalan edible animals, mentions the abundance of fauna: "These wild beasts are abundant in this land because of the many mountains."[35]

Based on the foregoing, it may be assumed that the lack of domestic animals as a source of protein was greatly compensated for by the abundant existing game. It is important to point out, furthermore, that the majority of the chroniclers mentioned in this chapter lived in Guatemala one or two centuries after the conquest, a period when the country was more populated and the area of cultivated land had expanded significantly.

The game animals mentioned by Ximénez were quite plentiful. Among the quadrupeds the following should be mentioned:

Deer (*Odocileus virginianus*)

> There are many in this land—small ones they call *viziz*, as well as big ones. Not only do many people eat them, but many other animals such as tigers, lions, and snakes. The Indians go out to catch the deer with their dogs by surrounding them, and restricting them to some place such as a river or a lake, and then jump in and catch them safely. They may also be tamed, as in Spain, and many of them are domesticated.[36]

Hog (Peccari)

> The hogs are unique and are commonly called wild bears. Some move in flocks through the fields, where they feed on fruits and wild roots, especially those that grow in swamps, where the hogs live much of the time, and in which they wallow and root like the hogs of Castilla. On the back of the hog is a little pouch called a navel, which is removed after killing the animal because otherwise it would infect the meat, which is lean and very tasty. When this animal is caught alive it may become so tame and domesticated that it walks behind the owner as if it were a dog.[37]

The *tacuatzín* (*Didelphis marsupialis*) was well described by Landa and mentioned earlier in this paper. Ximénez owned a *cotuza* (*Dasyprocta punctacta*), which "the Indians stole no doubt to eat, because it makes a very good dish." The armadillo (*Dasypus novencinctus fenestratus*) was "pursued by hunters, because it is very fine food." The water dog (*Lutra annectens*) had a "coat like velvet with which they make chairs and cushions and other things; the Indians also eat them." Finally there were many rabbits (*Sylvilagus floridanus*), "although they taste somewhat flat."[38]

Among the birds, Ximénez mentions the following: the *paujil* or *guan* (*Crax rubra*), "a bird one eats with great delight"; the turkey, called *chompipe* (*Meleagris gallopavo*) in Guatemala, was domesticated by the Indians, as mentioned earlier, but it also existed in the wild. There were also pigeons (*Columba liva*), which looked like the European partridges and quails, and numerous varieties of ducks which "are very good food, although somewhat heavy."[39]

Among the fish, Ximénez refers to the *guapote*, the *mojarra* (a sea fish), the *tepemechin*, the *pepesca*, "caught in the river of Amatitlán during the month of May, when they are full of eggs," and the *ilumina*, "small fish found in the rivers; there are many varieties of them, some as small as half of the little finger. If one had to count them it would be something infinite."[40]

Animals in Mayan Symbolism

In several of the codexes some dieties or anthropomorphic figures are represented carrying animals as an offering or as a symbol of their position.[41] In one of the *Codex Dresdensis*, for example, a woman is shown carrying in her hand a bowl with a fish, as a sign of offering; in her hair, as a headdress, she wears a coiled serpent, the symbolism of which is unknown. In the same codex, the God "K" appears carrying a bird in his right hand as an offering; with his left hand he is scattering the grains of sorcery or of fortune telling. It is interesting to observe in the same design a bowl with a bird, probably another offering, looking towards Yaxché, the tree of life. In another composition the God "A" appears, and in the bowl is a fish on a double *Kan* sign, which means food; another illustration shows the God "D," with the leg of a deer and the head of a bird in two bowls, the latter again with the *Kan*.

Another section of this codex shows a *tonalmatl* of fifty-two days divided into four equal groups, in each of which there is an edible animal, which could be a mammal, a reptile (iguana), or bird; these are probably to be offered to the gods, as again they are accompanied by the *Kan*.

The domestic dog was also used as an offering to the gods, for in the same codex a dog can be seen on top of a pyramid or *teocalli*.

How the Maya Hunted

The Indians were expert hunters. Accompanied by packs of hounds, large animals such as the deer and the hog were first hunted with the dart and the *ateatl* (dart-thrower) and later with bow and arrow. There were different varieties of arrows depending on their use: small animals and birds were hunted with popguns; for fishing the Indians used the net and the casting net, as well as the fish hook. In lagoons or small shallow rivers they used the bow and arrow, the latter with a special point. They also threw soporific drugs in the water, and when the fish came to the surface they were picked out by hand.[42] This practice had been used since the classic period, as may be seen from some archaeological pieces at Tikal. In any event it should be emphasized that the Maya did not fish in deep waters.

They were also expert in preparing hunting traps. Examples may be seen in the *Codex Tro-Cortesianus*.[43] In one a deer is caught by one leg by a rope tied to the branch of a tree; in another scene an armadillo has fallen into trap, and a bird, perhaps a turkey, has been caught with a net.

Apparently hunters and fishermen enjoyed great prestige within the social organization of Mayan communities, and special festivities were held annually in their honor. These had a twofold purpose: to ask and to thank the gods for good hunting or fishing; and to appease their wrath, which may have been provoked by the shedding of blood.[44]

The important festival was held in September, coinciding, according to Landa, with the day *Chuen* of the month of *Zip*. It was celebrated by priests, physicians, and sorcerers on consecutive days, followed by the hunters (*chaces*), and finally, the fishermen. The hunters met in

> the house of one of them, bringing their women with them, and the priests would come and throw out the devil. Once this had been done, they placed in the center the essentials for the sacrifice of incense, and new fire and blue pitch. The hunters then invoked the gods of the hunt, Acanum, Zuhuyzib, Zipitabai, and others, and distributed the incense, which they put on the brazier. While it burned, each hunter took out an arrow and the skull of a deer, which the other painted with the blue pitch. They then danced, holding the arrow and the skull in their hands; some pierced their ears and others their tongues, and through the holes they passed seven leaves of an herb they called *Ac*. After this, the priest and the officials of the feast offered their gifts, and, still dancing, the wine was poured and they got drunk until they were overcome by it.
>
> [The following day] the fishermen held their festivals in the same manner as the hunters, except they painted their fishing equipment and did not pierce their ears, but they performed a dance called *Chohom*.[45]

In February, the month of *Zac*, the priest fixed a similar feast day to that in the month of *Zip*, which "served to appease the gods' wrath against them and their farmlands."[46]

The hunted animals did not serve solely as food or as offerings to be sacrificed to the gods, they were also sold in the markets. Bernal Díaz del Castillo, when describing the market in Mexico City, mentions the sale of "hens, roosters with a wattle [turkeys], rabbits, hares, deer, mallards, dogs, and other things of this kind".[41]

Preparation and Consumption of Meats

The Indians prepared meat by broiling it over a fire or by stewing it with vegetables. "They make stews with vegetables and the meat of deer, wild and domestic birds, and fish, of which there are many, and they provide good nourishment."[48]

Díaz del Castillo, writing about "the manner and personality of the great Montezuma," describes the dishes eaten by the latter, and although his realm was beyond the original Mayan area, the cultural contacts of Middle America were so close that the tradition could be applied to the entire area.

> I heard they used to cook the flesh of very young boys, and as they had so many different stews made of so many things we did not notice if it was of human flesh or of other things, because every day they cooked hens, turkeys, pheasants, earth partridges, quails, domestic and wild ducks, deer, earth pigs, little cane birds, pigeons, hares, and rabbits, and many kinds of birds and things which grow in this land, of which there are so many I could not finish listing them.[49]

The Indians also had systems for preserving food, such as curing in smoke, which they used for the preparation of deer meat, the recipe for which, according to Gage, was to

> leave the deer covered with leaves for one week, until it begins to stink and becomes covered with maggots; they then take it home and cut it into pieces; later they boil it with an herb grown in this country that removes its bad smell, so they say, and makes the meat as tender and white as turkey. When it is half cooked they put the pieces in smoke for some time. When they are ready to eat it, they cook it again with a bit of red pepper.
>
> This is the venison of America that I have eaten on various occasions; however, I have not eaten much, not because it is not tasty, but because the memory of the maggots I had seen in it makes me nauseous.[50]

They also used the salting process as a means to preserve meat and fish. Finally they utilized smoking, drying, and salting methods for the preparation of the jerked or hung meat, which resulted in a kind of corned beef. This meat preservation process has been used by different cultures, and was known by the Spaniards before the discovery of America. This does not mean that the Indians did not know it, but it may be assumed that the Maya used it for the preservation of various kinds of meat.

FOOD: VEGETABLES

Growing and Consumption

The Maya grew and harvested a great variety of edible plants, many of which were adopted by the Western world and became basic foods in European diets. The potato, for example, was grown by the Indians of Peru, where, according to José de Acosta, it was "eaten fresh or cooked; a most tasty variety they make is a stew they call *locro*."[51] The potato was unknown to Central Americans, but they did consume various kinds of tubers such as sweet potatoes, yuccas, cassavas, and several kinds of yams.[52] The seed of the sweet potato was taken to Spain, where it was called *batata*, and

> it spread widely and grows very well, and thus it is a well-known food over there. Here they also grow in abundance and are important for the nourishment of men . . . . The yucca provides the daily bread of the islands of Barlovento. Although corn grows there, they do not have the habit of making bread out of it, which is much better than that made out of yucca, which they call *cazabe* . . . . To make the bread, the yucca is shredded and put in a press, where all the aqueous humor is removed from it. After it has been pressed they take some little pieces and put them in big flat pans or copper frying pans and place them on a fire where they seem to melt and stick together, forming a sort of pancake. It is very hard to eat, but if put into the soup, it puffs up well.[53]

The Indians grew several kinds of pumpkins or squash, "to obtain the seeds to make stews . . . and for several other purposes."[54] According to Ximénez:

> Over twenty varieties may be counted of all shapes and colors. They grow with such fierceness that if they find moist earth they produce all year round, and they turn into an almost infinite plant; it also produces roots in the earth and in this way spreads wherever it finds land, or is allowed to. There are others, which they call *tecomate* (bottle gourds), also in many shapes, which have many uses. In some hot places they are so big that two men cannot surround one. They make washbowls or platters out of these, cutting them in half, and painting them with great ingenuity.[55]

The *chipilín* was another shrub much utilized in the Mayan kitchen. It grew in "thickets, and sprouts by itself in the fields. Its leaves are stewed, but they are even eaten only cooked in water, without any seasoning, because they have a good taste and odor by themselves."[56]

The *pacaya*, a variety of *Chamaedorea*, a vegetable that "grows on small trees, usually becomes big and resembles the palmtree . . . it tastes like asparagus."[57]

Spices

Among the plants grown to give seasoning, aroma, and color to food were different varieties of chili (*ají*), "of which more than thirty may be counted." Among them "the *guaque* chili . . . *chamborote* . . . and another, medium-sized and very good, of which large crops are harvested, because it is the best. There is another one, short and wide, but very hot, and another thin one they call *chocolatl* . . . but of all, the hottest in these parts is a small one like a peppercorn, which they call *tempenchile*, so biting it seems like fire."[58]

Another pungent seasoning used by the Indians was the Tabasco pepper, described by Ximénez in the following manner:

> In this land there is a very good one, which subsitutes well for the lack of the one they call *Castilla*, because it has the same smell and is pungent. They grow on big trees, abundant in foliage, and of a great beauty. When the pepper is in little black clusters they pick it and dry it whole. The Indians of Verapaz and of Chiapa, where it is abundant, have many uses for it."[59]

To color the food red or orange they used annatto (*achiote*):

> The tree produces bunches of little flowers. The bristles sprout, and when they open up they are full of little seeds, covered by a fleshy dough, or putty, which is the annatto. When put in water it dissolves, and they then sieve it, remove the seeds, and boil that water until it thickens. It is used for dyes and for other purposes, especially for food; and it is very good for the urine."[60]

To give color to food they also used *achumico*, a "spice that grows on a tree and is picked in the same way as the annatto. It is used to give color, and some odor, to stews, and may be substituted frequently for saffron.[61]

FOOD: FRUITS

The land of the Maya was abundant in fruit trees. In the humid forests of Petén, *chico-sapota* grew wild, its fruit, usually like an orange, is one of the most delicious produced by nature. There are varieties of them: some big, others small, some round, others long. In San Salvador I have heard there is a kind where one *chico-sapota* is contained within another. This is one of the tastiest fruits this America produces in hot climates."[62]

Chewing gum was obtained from the same tree. For this purpose the stem was bled by making cuts in the bark; when the sap dried it turned into *chictli* or chewing gum. (This is the same method employed by modern chicle producers.)

The Maya utilized the wood of the *chico-sapota* tree to make doorheads for their temples and palaces, such as the famous *dintels* of Tikal, which are exquisitely carved.

Another important tree, called *ox* by the Maya, is now known as the "browse" (*ramón*) tree. It produces sweet and edible fruits; its seed provides an agreeable vegetable or, well dried and ground, becomes an edible flour; while its leaves are excellent fodder. According to Morley, "This tree must have been an important source of food in ancient times."[63]

Landa describes innumerable varieties of trees in the Yucatán, and expresses his thoughts as follows: "It makes one praise God with the prophet who says: 'Admirable it is, Lord, that Your Name is everywhere on earth,' for the multitude of trees in this land are all so different from ours that I have yet to see one I know." Next he refers to a series of native fruit trees of the region, which are briefly described by their Maya names, thus making it impossible to identify them in every case.[64]

Ximénez describes those fruits he considers most important:

> the *chico-sapota*, the *sapota*, and *annona* (custard apple). The plantain (*Musa paradisiaca*) is a tree that gives an exquisite fruit that is the nourishment of most of this America, especially in regions far away from trade ports. God has given it in such abundance it is unbelievable how much there is of this fruit everywhere. It is quite different from the plantain referred to in the Holy Scriptures, which is a big tree; this is not really a tree because its stem consists of joints that sprout from the root to the top, and in each joint is a big leaf. In this way it produces leaves from the heart until the last one that comes out is a bunch of plantains . . . of which there are many varieties; some are about half a *vara* and as thick as an arm . . . others are called Dominicans, of which there are three or four varieties; others are called bananas, of which there are also three or four varieties.[65]

The avocado (*Persea americana*) and the *jocotes* (*Spondias mombin*) "are usually considered exquisite. . . . Many call them plums because they are somewhat similar in shape and color; more than twenty varieties may be counted." Of the *matasano* (charlatan), (*Casimiroa tetramerica*), Ximénez says,

> although they have given this bad name to this fruit, which in New Spain is called white *sapota*, there is no reason for it, as everyone eats plenty of it and nobody dies from it. It is eaten mostly by poor people and the Indians, although some varieties are eaten by important people, because they have a delicious taste and smell.[66]

The *paterna, coginicuil* or *guajiniquil* (*Inga punctata*), "a hot country fruit, is similar to the carob bean . . . when the skin is opened, it is divided into little houses, each one having a somewhat hard seed covered by a very white and sweet little piece of pulp, which is what one eats." The *opuntia* or prickly pear (*Lemaireocereus eichlamii*) is "a fruit unique to this land . . . . Under this generic name there are many varieties—white, yellow, and purple." The *pitahaya* (*Lemaireocereus thurberii*) "grows attached to rocks, and its leaves are long, in the form of a triangle. . . . Its fruit is exquisite, of a very bright purple color." The *guayaba*, guava, (*Psidium guajava*) "is an abundant fruit in all the fields of this hot country," and the passion flower (*Hyperbaena guatemalensis*)

> is one of the most select because it is so nourishing and tasty . . . . It could not be less because its flower shows us our Redemption, as it contains the tools of the Most Holy Passion . . . we see in it very clearly the column in the center, the three nails, the five sores, the crown of thorns, and the twelve Apostles around it on twelve leaves . . . . [67]

BEE HONEY

Varieties of Honey Bees

Bee honey was used by the Maya for sweetening. Various species of bees existed, and the Maya of Yucatán cultivated at least two of them. Both, according to Landa, were smaller than European bees, and they had no sting. Ximénez, who apparently was a great beekeeper, studied the biology of the indigenous bees of Guatemala thoroughly. Like Landa, he identified two important varieties of honey-producing bees; one which, by antonomasia, he also called by the name of "bee"; the other was called *uscab* (honey mosquito) by the Indians and "young maid" by the Spaniards.[68] The former, Landa writes,

> resemble those in Spain in size, shape, and color, but they have no sting . . . they procreate in hollow trees . . . . in the center of which they put the young ones; their beehives are like those of the bees of Spain. With their wax these bees make containers or "potties," more or less the size of a pigeon egg, for the raw honey, which the Indians, who are very scientific about such things, rightfully call *raxcab*, green honey. They bring the nector in their mouths and place it in the potties until they are full, and then they cover them . . . . Next to one pottie they attach others in such a way as to make a sort of grape cluster . . . usually there are over thirty.[69]

The Indians then broke the potties and collected the honey.

The second variety of bees, described by Ximénez as "young maid," was smaller. They made their hives in the hollows of trees, between stones, or in the holes of mud walls and they produced honey "that is the best, the tastiest, and the most medicinal."

The Beekeepers and Their Festivals

The Maya domesticated these bees, and those responsible for taking care of them were given professional recognition. The assumption that honey was a favorite food among the Maya is proven by the fact that the beekeepers celebrated two religious feasts to beg the gods for larger crops of honey. The first was celebrated in the month of *Tzec* (mid-October), at which time they invoked the *bacabes*, especially *Hobnil*. They made many offerings and gave each of their gods a plate with a ball of incense in the center and figures made of honey painted around them. They usually ended the feast by drinking plenty of wine, which the owners of the hives provided in abundance. The second feast was celebrated in the month of *Mol* (early December) for the purpose of asking the gods to "provide flowers for the bees."[70]

In the last *Codex Tro-Cortesianus*, a section on bees contains essays on the raising, care, and, probably, rites related to this insect.[71]

COCOA AND CHOCOLATE

The Growing of Cocoa

Chocolate, the beverage of the Maya, was one of the greatest contributions of Middle America to Western culture. The Spanish conquistadores recognized immediately that chocolate was a delicious beverage, and soon introduced it to Europe, where, within a very few years, it gained great prestige, especially among the nobility. Gage, who on his trip through Central America, became an assiduous chocolate drinker, devotes an entire chapter of his book to a description of chocolate and its beneficial qualities.[72]

The word chocolate is derived from the ending *atle*, which in Nahuatl means water, and from the onomatopoeic word *choco*, the "choco-choco-choco" sound made by the beater in the mug wherein it is beaten to foam.

The main ingredient of chocolate is the grain inside the pod-shaped fruit of the cocoa tree, which was grown in the warm and humid climate of Campeche, Tabasco, and Belize, as well as in the mountainous Pacific watershed of Guatemala. In the Yucatán, due to the frequent droughts, it was grown only near the water reservoirs in caves.[73]

The cocoa tree was planted in the shade, and, to "defend it against the heat of the sun, they plant other trees they call the "mother of cocoa"; when these have grown sufficiently to cover the cocoa trees with their shade, they plant the cocoa plantations."[74] As described by Gage, this agricultural process in the colonial period is reminiscent of that of the Maya. The cocoa seeds had a twofold value: they were utilized as food and as a monetary unit.

Cocoa as Food: Chocolate

Landa tells us that in the Yucatán the Maya prepared a very tasty beverage made of ground corn and cocoa with which they celebrated their feasts. They also extracted from the cocoa "a grease that resembles butter, and with this and corn they made another tasty and popular beverage."[75] Ximénez confirms this when he informs us they extracted from the cocoa grains "a fat, that, upon cooling off, looks like very white wax . . . with which a very good beverage is made . . . it is also good to oint and refresh the back, and to oint the blisters that sometimes appear on the mouth, and on other parts."[76]

To prepare the beverage it was first necessary to make tablets or "bricks" by grinding cocoa grains that had been dried over fire on a stone carved especially for that operation, which the Indians called *metate*. Red-hot coals were placed under the *metate* to keep it hot, and in this way the cocoa acquired a pasty and moldable texture. The paste was then shaped into chunks on palmetto leaves and left in the shade to harden. The beverage was prepared with these chunks. According to Gage,

> the Indians prepare it by dissolving part of the chocolate with a few other ingredients . . . they beat it with a chocolate beater, and, after removing the greasy foam it forms, especially if the cocoa is old and has begun to mold, they put it on a plate, add sugar to the part from which they have removed the foam, and drink the chocolate completely cold. But a few people do resist it . . . and experience proves it is harmful and causes stomach aches, particularly in women.[77]

It should be remembered that Gage wrote during the Spanish rule, a period when the Indians were already using sugar as a sweetener; we assume that, if the Maya made sweetened chocolate in pre-Hispanic times, they had to do so with honey.

Cocoa as a Monetary Unit

It is known that the Indians used cocoa as a currency unit, especially in the markets, and that this custom extended into the colonial period. García Pelaez, in a report to Philip II on the province of Guatemala, indicates the value attached to cocoa as a currency, and gives the names of the different units the Indians used according to the number of cocoa grains: one *zontle* was equivalent to 400 grains; one *jiquipil* to twenty *zontles*; and one "load" to three *jiquipiles* (24,000 grains).[78]

SALT

Abundant salt mines existed in the Yucatán on a lagoon located very close to the sea. From the lagoon, where, Landa writes, "God created the best salt I have ever seen in my life," the Maya extracted salt at the end of the dry season. The inhabitants of the region had a monopoly on this exploitation, and every Indian was obliged to pay them some form of tribute; "all those who came for salt, rendered a small service, either the salt itself or product of their lands."[79]

The right to mine for salt had been required by a concession made to these settlers long ago by the lords of Mayapan. Yucatán thus became the largest salt-producing center in Central America; during a certain period of the colonial era, salt was exported to Mexico, Guatemala, Honduras, and Cuba.[80]

Some rock-salt mines also existed on the central high plateau of Guatemala, such as the Chixoy Valley,[81] but this was not as valuable as the sea salt, which was marketed throughout the entire Mayan world. In some regions where there was no salt, it was produced "from ashes they make from palm trees, which they burn and boil . . . the resulting sieved lye makes a very loose salt. Thus in those parts . . . where the people avail themselves of this industry, the men are bloated. There is no doubt that one of the most necessary things for the maintenance of human life is salt.[82]

DAILY LIFE AND THE HABITUAL FOOD

Early rising was a habit with the Maya. First the woman got up between four and six in the morning to light the fire and heat the *tortillas*, the beans, and the *atole* (corn-flour beverage) with pepper, which constituted their breakfast.[83] (The *tortillas* were probably left over from the previous day and reheated.) Then the men left for the field to work on their corn plantations, to cut lumber, and to perform other farming tasks. They took with them a ball of *pozole* (brew) the size of an apple, wrapped in a plantain leaf. *Pozole* was corn dough, *zacan*, boiled and hardened, which when dry lasted several months. If the Indian felt hungry, he interrupted his work and took a "pellet and dissolved it in a bowl of cold water made from the skin of a fruit."[84] Landa refers to the *jicara* (chocolate cup), or *puch* in Maya. When the dough was dissolved it nourished the worker for the rest of the morning until he returned home.

In the meantime the women took care of the home. They were, in Landa's words,

> very thrifty workers, because they are responsible for most of the tasks that support their households; for the education of their children; and for the payment of tributes . . . in addition to all this, if necessary they sometimes carry the burden of tilling and sowing their fields. They are marvelous farmers, keeping vigil at night during the time they have left after serving their families, and going to the market to buy and sell their produce. They raise and sell their own birds, and those from Castilla,* and use the feathers for making smart clothes . . . they also raise domestic animals, including the roe deer, which become so tame they never go away to the mountains.[85]

A great part of the Mayan women's time was spent preparing the corn to make *tortillas* and *pozole*; this was probably "one the most important activities of a Mayan woman's life—second only to bearing and raising her children.[86]

The most important meal, according to a sixteenth century narrative, transcribed by Morley, was the evening meal:

> An hour before sunset it was their custom to make certain tortillas of the said dough. On these they supped, dipping them in certain dishes of crushed peppers, diluted with a little water and salt. Alternately with this they ate certain boiled beans of the land, which are black. They call them *buul*, and the Spanish, *frijoles*. This was the only time they ate during the day, for at other times they drank the dissolved dough mentioned above.[87]

This main meal also consisted of stews of fresh meat, salted fish, or venison. Once in a while they would eat the meat of *tzimin* (tapir), *zub* (armadillo), *ac* (turtle), and *baclam* (manatee). In addition to the corn and the beans, there were also vegetables such as squash or pumpkin and *güisquil* or *chayote*.

The men did not usually eat with the women, who served them on the

---

* The Spaniards had brought birds over by the time Landa wrote his book.

floor or, at best, using a mat as a table. After eating they washed their hands and mouths. The women ate after the men had gone back to work or were resting.[88]

The family went to bed as soon as it became dark. Before withdrawing, however, the women smothered the fire to keep it alive until the next day, and put the remaining *tortillas* in a *col* made out of a pumpkin shell.

But not everything was routine in the life of the Maya: they had their feasts and celebrations, when their feeding habits changed and "they ate, sitting in groups of twos or fours, and after they had eaten, the cupbearers brought some big drinking tubs until everybody got into a scuffle."[89] Their customary alcoholic beverage was made of honey diluted in water, a kind of hydromel or mead fortified with the root or bark of the *balche* tree,[90] which made the wine strong and very malodorous. If lords or important people attended these banquets, the menu consisted of broiled fowl, *tortillas*, and a cocoa beverage. They offered what they had so generously "that many times they spent on a banquet what it took them many days to earn."[91]

CHILD CARE AND FEEDING

The gift of fertility was highly valued among the ancient Maya and their descendents. Furthermore, they loved children dearly and each birth was greeted with great happiness. Each family wanted many children and a women who did not have any beseeched her idols for them with gifts and prayers.

The Maya-Quiché Indians also offered sacrifices to have children, and in cases of sterility they extracted blood from various parts of their bodies, made promises, sacrificed birds, resorted to sorcery, and sought the advice of their priests. The latter,

> diabolical men, responded by saying that because of their sins the gods did not permit them to have sons or daughters, and sent them to do penance . . . usually by separating a husband and wife for a period of forty or fifty days; not letting them eat anything with salt; prescribing a diet of dry bread or corn. . . . The desire to have children was so great that nothing that the priests ordered them to do, grave as it might be, seemed difficult; and thus they named the first child born to them after the idol, who was dedicated to the day of the birth.[92]

The woman took care of herself during her pregnancy and was put on a special diet; although she continued to perform all her daily household chores, she avoided certain tasks, especially work in the field. The preparation of food continued to be her main occupation, and during moments of leisure she wove blankets to cover her future child. When the time for confinement arrived the family resorted to the sorcerers, who "made the parents believe their lies and placed under their bed an idol of a demon called Ixchael, who, they said, was the goddess of pregnancy and of confinement."[93] The newborn child was bathed immediately.

Four or five days later the Maya of Yucatán began the process of artificially flattening the cranium. This practice consisted in tying two flat boards to the child's head, one over the fontanel and the other at the back of the head. They were left in that position for a few days, and when they were removed the head was flattened and the forehead depressed. This cranial deformity, considered a sign of beauty by the ancient Maya, was almost universal, particularly among members of high social classes.

The Maya-Quiché Indians of the high plateau of Guatemala did not practice this custom; instead, when a child was born they sacrificed a bird or sent it to a priest to offer to the gods in the child's behalf. The relatives then had a series of parties. When they washed the child in a fountain or river, they offered new sacrifices of incense and birds. They also offered all the utensils and instruments the woman had used during the confinement. Later

> they drew lots to see which day would be propitious to cut off the umbilical cord, and on that day they placed the cord on an ear of corn, and, with an unused knife, cut if off and threw the knife into a bowl as a blessed object. They then took the kernels off the corn and planted it. The kernels were ground and the first pap was given to the child.[94]

The children were breast-fed from birth until they were three or four years old. Indian women had very rich milk because they drank a hot corn beverage, and therefore they were good nurses. Even today, beverages made with corn are reputedly galactogenous and Indian women drink them frequently.[95]

The abundant supply of milk and the care given by the mothers caused the Mayan children to develop satisfactorily from a nutritional point of view. There is no doubt that the extended period of suckling had a favorable effect. The Maya were unaware of other sources of milk for human feeding, for they had no milk-producing domestic animals. They did recognize the fact that human milk could be used to feed other animal species, however, and that it was an essential factor in the feeding of the newborn animal. This is evidenced by Landa's statement that the Indian women fed the roe deer with human milk.[96] Furthermore, the Maya utilized wet nurses as substitutes for the mother in child feeding.

Although the Maya of Yucatán apparently had no ritual or festivity at the time of weaning, Maya-Quiché families threw a big party to which they invited relatives and neighbors. A sacrifice was made to the gods indicated for that day, and the family then gave the child the "first pap" prepared with the corn flour obtained from the ritual grains at the time the cord was cut off.[97] From that time on the child ate the same food as the rest of the family.

COMMENTS

Habitual Diet and Nutritional Value

The information available is far too incomplete to enable us to divide the foods into their nutritional components and thereby to determine the native Mayan diet; but it does give us a general idea of their habitual diet and its composition.

A great lack of nourishment is a prevailing cultural feature in Mayan society. The Indians did not eat for pleasure but out of need, and their diet was frugal and simple, although varied.[98] The Mayan was thin and muscular, lacking any unnecessary adipose tissue; obesity and other disorders caused by overeating were unknown.

The feeding practices of modern Guatemalan Indians are not much different than those of their forefathers, except in terms of variety. The diet continues to be frugal, consisting primarily of corn and beans, due to the poverty in which our present Indian peasant population lives.[99] The varied diet of the ancient Mayan Indian was due to the availability of game. Today there are no longer any game animals, and, with the exception of some fowl and pigs, domestic animals are scarce. This situation is largely due to a lack of pasture land, and to the fact that the Indian cannot afford to feed animals with the grains he needs for his own nourishment. It could be said that animal feeding is competing with human feeding.

The ancient Maya's diet was balanced nutritionally. He obtained his energy primarily from corn and secondarily from beans and other foods, particularly roots and tubers. Corn alone, however, supplied the greatest part of the calories the Maya needed. Cocoa, although it has great energy value due to its fat content, could not be considered as a usual source of calories because its consumption was restricted to the ruling oligarchies and other high social groups. Most of the people consumed it only on certain festive occasions when chocolate was served as a beverage of great prestige. Neither can the importance of honey be determined as a source of energy, since no precise information exists regarding its production and consumption. We know it was used in the preparation of beverages, but the amount consumed is unknown. It is quite probable, however, that due to the limitations of the beehives only a small amount of honey was part of the daily diet.

Protein in the Maya's nutrition was provided to a large extent by corn and beans. While the protein in corn is of a relatively poor quality, it improves considerably when combined with that in beans. The optimum corn:bean ratio needed to achieve total supplementary effect was not reached by the normal diet of the Indian.[100] It is probable that the difference today is the same that existed in the past, as the technique for sewing the corn was and is closely linked to that of beans.

This deficiency in high quality protein was overcome by the ancient Maya through the consumption of game animals and fish, as well as domestic animals. The large variety of vegetables and fruits provided them with the carotene and vitamins A and C not present in the other foods.

Diet and Nutritional Diseases

The Maya's habitual diet, as described here, supplied all the required nutrients for a balanced diet; if nutritional diseases existed, they were probably of minimum epidemiological significance and limited to sporadic cases, or to small epidemic outbursts under certain specific conditions, for example, during famines.[101]

The only serious nutritional problem, due to its great prevalence and secondary consequences, was the endemic goiter caused by a deficiency of iodine. This condition persisted until recent times: it has only been in the last few years that it has been virtually eradicated, thanks to iodized salt.

That goiter was recognized by the Maya is evidenced in clay figures, where the swelling produced in the throat by the thyroid may be easily seen, and by the fact that there was a word for goiter in the Mayan and Mayan-Quiché languages.[102]

It was also described by chroniclers of the colonial period, particularly by Gage when writing of his trip from Chiapas to Guatemala. Upon entering the village of Sacapulas,

> in a grove near the water I met the Prior of Sacapulas himself with a large committee of Indians, who were awaiting me with a cup of chocolate. At first I was somewhat shocked by the Prior, who had a terrible . . . pouch all around his neck, which hung down to his shoulders and chest . . . thereby lifting his head in such a way that he could hardly look to any other side but at the sky. During the course of our conversation he told me that he had been suffering

from the disease for ten years, and that the water from that river was the cause
. . . . This made me lose my love for the river . . . and I resolved not to stay in
that place as long as I had thought I would for fear the water would mark me
for life . . . . When I arrived in the village I discovered many men and women
with pouches on their throats like the poor Prior, which almost made me lose
the desire to drink the chocolate made with that water or to eat anything
washed with it. But the Prior encouraged me by telling me it did little harm,
and only when one drank it cold; wherefore I resolved to stay there four or five
days because the Prior . . . promised to teach me the Indian language.[103]

Protein-calorie malnutrition in children, which today exists in almost all traditional peasant cultures of the world, was probably not a serious nutritional problem among the precolonial Maya. The evidence in favor of this hypothesis is based on the fact that the Indians had a repertoire of names for their most common diseases and symptoms. A list of these diseases does not contain any word for protein-calorie malnutrition or any of the characteristics of the disease;[104] if it had been prevalent, the Maya probably would have had a name for it.

We do not wish to state categorically that protein-calorie malnutrition did not exist; we believe it did, but only as a sporadic disease. Two factors may be responsible for this low prevalence: first, the practice of extended breast feeding, and, second, the gradual introduction to the family diet when the child was still receiving mother's milk, that is, until the age of three to four. Let us remember, furthermore, that the habitual family diet, as mentioned earlier, was better balanced than it is today, and was rich in animal proteins. The chief nutritional demands of the growing child were satisfied with more and better proteins than the Indian child now receives.

Famines

The fact that nutritional diseases, with the exception of goiter, were not of great significance does not mean the Maya had no serious adversities in terms of food. Famines occurred repeatedly, and all Indian manuscripts refer directly or indirectly to episodes of this nature. Such an event is referred to in the *Memorial de Tecpán-Atitlán*, when, as a consequence of a great frost that occurred in the Cakchiquel kingdom, the entire population suffered from hunger.

There was great hunger caused by an intense cold which destroyed the sown fields in the month of *Uchum*, and all the crops were lost . . . . our forefathers said all food was finished. Oh, my children . . . . the people cannot endure the sufferings from that great hunger.[105]

We find similar statements by other writers,[106] and Landa mentions the occurrence of two famines at the time the first Spaniards arrived.[107]

The lack of a sufficient agricultural surplus, due to the Indians' predominantly subsistence farming, and defects in their ability to store food were the responsible factors for the starvation that occurred during these famines. Mayan agricultural techniques were relatively primitive, and subsistence agriculture did not allow food to be conserved, except for very limited periods of time. The lack of quadruped animals that could be domesticated and used for agricultural tasks and for transportation were decisive factors in their agricultural feeding potential. They did not know the plow, but they did invent a similar implement that also required manpower.[108]

All these factors contributed to the fact that any uncontrollable phenomenon caused serious agricultural calamities and consequent famines. For that reason such disasters were considered supernatural, and the Indians either raised them to the status of deities, in the case of rain, which they symbolized in the god, Chac, or were considered a supernatural whim, in which case they saw themselves forced to offer sacrifices to appease the wrath of their gods or to ask them for favors.

The ancient Maya were industrious, and in spite of temporary famines, which technologically underdeveloped cultures are bound to have, they lived in a prodigal land where their culture had taken deep roots in an open symbiosis with the environment.

In conclusion, let me quote the great contemporary Maya expert, Sylvanus G. Morley, as he interprets the Mayan civilization:

> ... nature's richest gift to man was maize—the Maya staff of life—without which they never could have developed their highly distinctive culture, the most brilliant aboriginal civilization of the New World. And if we bear constantly in mind the fact that from three-fourths to five-sixths of everything the average Maya eats, even today, is corn in one form or another, and that their culture was based directly upon, and derives straight from, agriculture as applied to the cultivation of corn, we shall have learned the most basic fact about the Maya civilization.[109]

NOTES

1. J. Antonio Villacorta, transl., *Popul Vuh* (Guatemala: Tipografía Nacional, 1934).
2. Sylvanus G. Morley, *The Ancient Maya* (Palo Alto: Stanford University Press, 1946).
3. P.C. Mangelsdorf and J.W. Cameron, "Western Guatemala; a Secondary Center of Origin of Cultivated Maize Varieties," *Botanical Museum Leaflets* (Harvard University) 10 (1942): 217-52.

4. Morley, *Ancient Maya* (See note 2).
5. Francisco Ximénes, *História Natural del Reino e Guatemala* (1722; reprint ed., Guatemala: Editorial "José Pinada Ibarra," 1957).
6. Morley, *Ancient Maya* (See note 2).
7. Ibid.
8. Ibid.
9. Fray Diego de Landa, *Relación de las Cosas de Yucatán* (1560; reprint ed., México: Editorial Porrua S.A., 1959).
10. Morley, *Ancient Maya* (See note 4).
11. Ximénes, *História Natural* (See note 5).
12. Michael D. Coe, *The Maya* (New York: Frederick A. Praeger, 1969).
13. Landa, *Yucatán* (See note 9).
14. Tomas Gage, *Nueva Relación que Contiene los Viajes de Tomas Gage en la Nueva España* (1838; reprint ed. Guatemala: Tipografía Nacional 1946).
15. Landa, *Yucatán* (See note 9).
16. Ricardo Bressani, A.T. Valiente, and Carlos Tejada, "All-Vegetable Protein Mixtures for Human Feeding. VI. The Value of Combinations of Lime-Treated Corn and Cooked Black Beans," *Journal of Food* (S.A.) 27 (1962): 394-400.
17. Ximénes, *História Natural* (See note 5).
18. Francisco Antonio de Fuentes y Guzman, *Recordación Florida. Códice del Siglo XVII (1690)* (Guatemala: Tipografía Nacional, 1932).
19. Gage, *Los Viajes* (See note 14).
20. Ximénes, *História Natural* (See note 5).
21. Bernabé Cobo, *História del Nuevo Mundo (XVII century)* Cited in J. Garcia Mercabel, *Lo Que España Llevó a América* (n.p.: Tauros, Ediciones S.A., 1959).
22. Bernal Díaz del Castillo, *História Verdadera de la Conquista de la Nueva España* (n.p.: n.p., 1906).
23. Landa, *Yucatán* (See note 9).
24. Ximénes, *História Natural* (See note 5).
25. J. Antonio Villacorta and Carlos A. Villacorta, *Códices Mayas: Dresdensis, Peresianus y Tro-Cortesianus* (Guatemala: Tipografía Nacional, 1933).
26. Coe, *The Maya* (See note 12).
27. Landa, *Yucatán* (See note 9).
28. Ibid.
29. Ibid.
30. Ibid.
31. Ibid.
32. Ibid.
33. Ibid.
34. Ibid.
35. Ximénes, *História Natural* (See note 5).
36. Ibid.
37. Ibid.
38. Ibid.
39. Ibid.
40. Ibid.
41. Villacorta and Villacorta, *Códices Mayas* (See note 25).
42. Coe, *The Maya* (See note 12).
43. Villacorta and Villacorta, *Códices Mayas* (See note 25).
44. Landa, *Yucatán* (See note 9).
45. Ibid.
46. Ibid.
47. Díaz, *Nueva España* (See note 22).
48. Landa, *Yucatán* (See note 9).

49. Díaz, *Nueva España* (See note 22).
50. Gage, *Los Viajes* (See note 14).
51. José de Acosta, *História Natural y Moral de las Indias (Vida Religiosa de los Indios)* (1590, reprint ed., México: Universidad Nacional Autónoma de México, 1963).
52. Morley, *Ancient Maya* (See note 2).
53. Ximénes, *História Natural* (See note 5).
54. Landa, *Yucatán* (See note 9).
55. Ximénes, *História Natural* (See note 5).
56. Ibid.
57. Ibid.
58. Ibid.
59. Ibid.
60. Ibid.
61. Ibid.
62. Ibid.
63. Morley, *Ancient Maya* (See note 2).
64. Landa, *Yucatán* (See note 9).
65. Ximénes, *História Natural* (See note 5).
66. Ibid.
67. Ibid.
68. Ibid.
69. Landa, *Yucatán* (See note 9).
70. Ibid.
71. Villacorta and Villacorta, *Códices Mayas* (See note 25).
72. Gage, *Los Viajes* (See note 14).
73. Coe, *The Maya* (See note 12).
74. Gage, *Los Viajes* (See note 14).
75. Landa, *Yucatán* (See note 9).
76. Ximénes, *História Natural* (See note 5).
77. Gage, *Los Viajes* (See note 14).
78. Francisco de Paula García Pelaez, *Memorias para la História del Antigua Reino de Guatemala*, 3rd ed. (Guatemala: Tipografía Nacional, 1968).
79. Landa, *Yucatán* (See note 9).
80. Ibid.
81. Coe, *The Maya* (See note 12).
82. Ximénes, *História Natural* (See note 5).
83. Landa, *Yucatán* (See note 9).
84. Ibid.
85. Ibid.
86. Morley, *Ancient Maya* (See note 2).
87. Ibid.
88. Landa, *Yucatán* (See note 9).
89. Ibid.
90. Victor W. Von Hagen, *The Ancient Sun Kingdoms of the Americas* (Cleveland: World Publishing, 1957).
91. Landa, *Yucatán* (See note 9).
92. Francisco Ximénes, *História de la Provincia de San Vicente de Chiapa y Guatemala* (Guatemala Editorial "José Pineda Ibarra," 1965).
93. Landa, *Yucatán* (See note 9).
94. Ximénes, *História de la Provincia* (See note 92).
95. Carlos Martínez Durán, *Las Ciencias Médicas en Guatemala. Origen y Evolución*, 3rd ed. (Guatemala: Editorial Universitario, 1964).
96. Landa, *Yucatán* (See note 9).
97. Ximénes, *História de la Provincia* (See note 92).

98. Landa, *Yucatán* (See note 9).
99. Martínez Durán, *Ciencias Médicas* (See note 95).
100. Bressani, Valiente, and Tejada, "Human Feeding" (See note 16).
101. Moisés Béhar, "Food and Nutrition of the Maya before the Conquest and at the Present Time," in *Biomedical Challenges Presented by the American Indian* (Washington: Pan American Health Organization, scientific publication No. 165, 1968); and Martínez Durán, *Ciencias Médicas* (See note 95).
102. Stephan F. Borhegyi and Nevin S. Scrimshaw, "Evidence for Pre-Coloumbian Goiter in Guatemala," *American Antiquity* 23 (1957): 174-76.
103. Gage, *Los Viajes* (See note 14).
104. Martínez Durán, *Ciencias Médicas* (See note 95).
105. J. Antonio Villacorta, transl. *Memorial de Tecpán-Atitlán. Anales de los Cakchiqueles* (Guatemala: Tipografía Nacional, 1936).
106. Alfredo Barrera Vasques and Silvia Rendón, transl. *El Libro de los Libros de Chilam Balam* (México: Fondo de Cultura Económica, 1965).
107. Landa, *Yucatán* (See note 9).
108. Antonio De Herrera, *História General de los Hechos de los Castellanos en las Islas i Tierra Firme del Mar Oceano*, 5 vols., 2nd ed. (Madrid: n.p., 1726-30); and García Peláez, *Memorias* (See note 78).
109. Morley, *Ancient Maya* (See note 2).

DISCUSSANT:

E. Croft Long

Dr. Tejada has undertaken a major study of the nutrition and feeding practices of the people of Central America, and his presentation concerning the habits of the Indians in pre-Columbian times deserves the most careful attention. The point I wish to emphasize is not only the practical importance of this study to historians, but to all those concerned with nutrition. While it could be described as a historical review, to those concerned with improving the nutritional status of the people of Central America it could with equal accuracy be called an operational research document on nutrition.

In Guatemala at present about 870,000 children are under the age of five, comprising around 20 percent of the total population. INCAP's studies have shown that some 80 percent of these children—approximately 700,000—are malnourished to some degree, and that 44,000 suffer from Grade III malnutrition on the Gomez Scale. The Indians, who comprise something over 55 percent of the population, have a life expectancy at birth of about forty-five years. Some twenty-two different languages are spoken by the Guatemalan Indians, many of whom do not speak Spanish.

Now if we combine these data with the fact that 36 percent of the people live in communities of less than 500, we see at once the problems that face those interested in improving the nutritional status of the people—problems related to numbers and to accessibility or inaccessibility. The relationship between food and disease is an ancient and fundamental belief; it was observed by Bishop Díego de Landa, who described the way in which foods were classified according to a type of physiological principle that distinguished them as being "hot" or "cold": foods were recognized as being more or less in one or the other of these categories. Hot foods, for example, included honey, coffee, and beef; cold foods included turkey, rice, papaya, and pork. In relation to sickness it was believed that weakness and instability were due to eating excessively cold foods, and that fever, for example, was due to eating too many hot foods. The treatment of these conditions was a logical principle, which provided that cold foods be eaten for "hot" diseases, and vice versa. Any attempt to change nutritional practices without taking into account such beliefs would obviously be unsuccessful.

Dr. Tejada also pointed out the traditional role of corn in the culture of the Indian people; and of the symbolism of corn as seen repeatedly in stellae, painting, pottery, and Mayan writings in the *Popul Vuh*. Likewise you see ritual regulating the planting and harvesting of the corn crop.

These beliefs were fundamental and at the root of all nutrition education, especially when we bear in mind the fact that, as Dr. Tejada has pointed out, maize provided one of the major protein sources. Similar studies could I think be usefully developed in the field of agricultural practices and traditions, because that type of study would provide the logical basis for penetrating the Indian communities, which are resistant to modernization. The cultural roots of 2,000 years cannot be eliminated, but they can be utilized to disseminate the new knowledge and experience we now have at our disposal.

Dr. Tejada's paper raises a number of questions, among which is whether nutritional experts take advantage of this hot or cold theory of disease. I wonder whether these beliefs he has described to us have changed, and whether those nutritional practices and beliefs perhaps played any role in the decline of the Mayan empire. I wonder also whether there is information on the beliefs and habits of other Indian groups such as those in Costa Rica and in Nicaragua. Also, of course, it would be interesting to hear about food prejudices among the Ladino population, because of the high rate of malnourishment among this group.

In addition, we wonder how the nutrition practices of the Maya of pre-Columbian times relate to the present. Dr. Guerra yesterday pointed out the important role of breast-feeding of infants because of the lack of animal protein, but the Maya did have access to turkeys, which they domesticated. Dr. Tejada has pointed out that they had venison in Yucatan, in particular, and we wonder if the eating of sacrificial victims might have been motivated by nutritional rather than by ritualistic trends. These are some of the thoughts that Dr. Tejada's paper has provoked.

HISTORICAL SYNTHESIS OF MEDICAL EDUCATION IN MEXICO

Jaime Mendiola Gomez

If the arrival of the Spaniards in Mexico signified for the Indians the destruction of their culture, the newcomers did bring with them some positive aspects of European civilization. An example is the work of a group of Franciscan monks who arrived in Mexico on 14 May 1524. Headed by Fray Martín de Valencia, the monks were entrusted with the mission of evangelizing the Indians of the recently discovered New World.

In 1536 they founded the Imperial College of Santa Cruz in Santiago-Tlaltelolco, now located in the heart of Mexico City. Here the natives were taught Latin, philosophy, music, reading, writing, and rhetoric. They also received instruction in medicine, and it was from this college that the first physicians of New Spain emerged, among them Martín de la Cruz, the Indian author of the first book on pharmacology edited in America, the *Badian Codex,* so-called by its translator, Juan Badiano.

Before the arrival of the Spaniards the teaching of medicine had been totally empirical. The Aztecs passed down their knowledge from generation to generation, as they did their expertise in handcrafts. Tlamatiliztemach-tiani, the master, introduced his descendents to the secrets of *ticiotl* (medicine), instructing them in diseases and their cure, and the use of plants and animals in the treatment of diseases that were believed to be caused by the gods, among whom Tzapotlatenan, Xipe, Tetzcatlipoca, Tlaltecuin, and Quetzalcoatl stood out.

Although the Franciscans initiated the teaching of medicine in Mexico, it was not until 21 September 1551, by royal decree of King Charles V, that

Don Antonio de Mendoza, first viceroy of New Spain, founded the Royal Pontifical University of Mexico, "as it has been requested that a university or school of all sciences be founded in the said Mexico City, where all the natives and the sons of Spaniards be taught matters of our Holy Catholic faith and other sciences [sic]."

The University of Mexico was a true copy of European universities, and it had the same defects: the scant scientific basis of medicine at that time, its lack of popularity, and the influence of the beliefs of the Middle Ages were all reflected in that institution. The first medical professorship was created by the rector, Bernabé Valdés de Cárcamo in 1579. The first medical course was initiated on 7 January 1579, according to some historians, and on 7 November 1582 according to others. The course was called "beginning medicine" *(Prima de Medicina)*, and the professorship was granted to Juan de la Fuente.

Thus, some fifty years after the initial instruction given by the Franciscans, the teaching of medicine received its first official sanction at the university level, coinciding with the outbreak of a series of epidemics. Father Mendieta tells us that epidemics dated from the time of the arrival of Pánfilo de Narváez in 1520 until the end of the sixteenth century, the most serious being measles and smallpox.

The teaching of medicine was to undergo a slow evolution. Twenty years after the first course was created came a second one, "prelude to medicine"; this professorship was granted to Juan de Plascencia in 1598. A third course, anatomy and surgery, was not begun until 1620; the professorship was initially filled by Francisco de Urieta, and later by Rodrigo Muñóz. A royal ordinance of Philip III decreed that candidates for the bachelor (first) degree had to complete all three courses. The professorship in anatomy and surgery was granted, not without difficulties, to Muñóz, who was forced to appeal to the court because he was expected to have a special degree in surgery, which he considered improper and unnecessary "because he had graduated as a Bachelor, a Licensed Practitioner and Doctor from the School of Medicine."

Beginning medicine, "related to the healthy man," took four years, and used very old-fashioned textbooks: *The Prognostics, Epidemics,* and *Aphorisms* of Hippocrates. Prelude to medicine was also covered in four years and used, in addition to the foregoing works, Avicena's *De Agritudinibus, De Causis,* and *De Accidentibus*. The textbooks used for methods and practice of medicine, a course created some time after anatomy and surgery, and taught by Francisco de Urieta, were Galileo's *De Morbis Curandi, De Arte Curativa ad Glaucomen,* and *De Medica Artis Constitutione,* as well as his texts on anatomy and surgery.

The methods of instruction followed the European pattern: theoretical teaching based on the foregoing works, which at that time had been in existence for twenty centuries. The students had no contact with patients. The skeleton was studied once a month. The first autopsy took place in 1646; it was not repeated until 1651 because autopsies were permitted only on the corpses of persons who had been sentenced to death.

In general, medicine at the end of the sixteenth century was not considered a very important career, and above all it was unpopular—the refuge of backward students whose professors were the lowest paid in the university.

It should be mentioned, however, that important works were produced during that period: *Opera Medicinalia* by Francisco Bravo (1570); *Summary and Compilation of Surgery with a Method for Bleeding, Very Useful and Beneficial* by Alonso López (1578); *Brief Treatise on Medicine*, by García de Farfán; and *Brief Treatise on Surgery, and Knowledge and Cause of Certain Diseases* by Augustín Farfán.

At the end of the sixteenth century Francisco Hernández, First Physician of the Indies, arrived in Mexico. He was entrusted by Philip II with the task of compiling information about Mexican flora and fauna and Indian medicine. The results of his investigations were published in the seventeen-volume *De Historia Plantarum Nova Hispaniae.*

During the first third of the seventeenth century the University of Mexico went through an era of spiritual and material progress, with the incorporation by then of the "Gentlemen of the Royal Court" and members of the Holy Inquisition, as well as members of such religious orders as the Metropolitan Church, Augustinians, and Dominicans. Among the professors were Diego Martínez de los Ríos, professor of beginning medicine, "who had a salary of 500 pesos a year," Damián Gonzáles Cueto, professor of prelude to medicine, "with a salary of 300 pesos a year," Juan Sotelo de Betanzos, and Francisco de Urieta.

By 1640 the School of Medicine had fourteen students and five professors: Manuel de Sosa, Domingo Arias, Diego de Magaña, Lucas de Cárdenas, and Matías del Salcedo. In a way, the appointment of Sosa constituted an imposition on the part of the viceroy, Marqués de Villena, who ordered the faculty to appoint Sosa professor of beginning medicine. While this was considered coercion and an affront to the dignity of the university, the order was obeyed, although not as "a voluntary act."

In 1651 competitive examinations were given for the post of professor of introduction to medicine. The results favored Arias, who assumed the professorship on 5 November. This post again became vacant upon Arias's death, but new examinations were not given and Magaña took the post on

20 April 1652. At the death of Fernández Osorio, the professorship of introduction to medicine was assumed by Gerónimo de Ortíz on the viceroy's recommendation. When Magaña died his post was taken by Méndez de Olaeta.

The imposition of professors of medicine by the viceroys of New Spain was followed by the somewhat unusual procedure of the election of professors by the students, and it was in this manner that Nicolás Méndez de Ola, and, later, Juan de Torres Moreno, obtained their appointments.

The year 1680 is significant because for the first time a surgeon was appointed as professor of anatomy: the post was granted to José García by Viceroy Conde de Paredes, who ordered the faculty "to have him as a Professor of Anatomies made and to be made at the said Royal University and Hospitals of this Court."

As a result of the knowledge and experience of Mexican and Spanish doctors, the following works were published during the seventeenth century: *True Surgery, Medicine and Astrology* by Juan de Barrios (1607); *Place, Nature and Properties of the City of Mexico. Rains and Winds to Which It Is Subject and Climates of the Year* by Diego Cisneros (1618); *The Treasure of Medicine for Various Diseases* by the Honorable Gregorio López (1672); and *Principia Medicinae, Epitome et Tortius Humani Corporis Fabrica* by Osorio y Peralta.

OFFICE OF ROYAL PHYSICIANS

The first Office of Royal Physicians, established at the end of the sixteenth century, was charged with maintaining a high level of professional standards among physicians and those in similar professions. The institution was integrated by three examiners with the titles of royal physician, a lawyer, a notary, and three assistant examiners. Their principal task was to supervise professional examinations for physicians, surgeons, pharmacists, and phlebotomists. A secondary task was to verify licenses and control the drugs sold to the public. This body was frequently consulted by the viceroy, especially on problems relating to medicine and public health.

To be eligible to take the examination to qualify as a surgeon, each candidate had to file with the Office of Royal Physicians a copy of his baptismal certificate, a notarized statement that he had undergone a five-year apprenticeship with a surgeon, that he was legally married, that he was a legitimate child, that his parents were Christian and Spanish, with no Moorish, Jewish, Chinese, or Negro blood, and that he had never been punished by the Inquisition.

The examination consisted of several theoretical questions concerning surgery, and a practical examination of four patients whose diseases had to be diagnosed and the proper treatment prescribed. The candidate then had to take an oath "to defend the mystery of the Immaculate Conception of the Virgin Mary, to observe Royal orders, and to give free treatment to the poor."

Persons who desired to practice medicine in New Spain could aspire to three university degrees: bachelor, licensee, and physician. To obtain the bachelor degree a candidate first had to have an arts degree, for which he had to take several courses at the university, including beginning medicine, prelude to medicine, anatomy and surgery, astronomy and mathematics, and methods of medicine. The arts examination consisted of sixteen questions by eight examiners, supervised by the rector. At the conclusion of the examination the candidate made an act of faith, took an oath on the bylaws of the university, and promised to defend the belief in the virginity of Mary.

To practice medicine a bachelor was required to have had two years of practice at the school, and to have taken an examination before the Office of the Royal Physicians. Once he had passed he was automatically prohibited from using a knife, a sword, or any other weapon.

To obtain a licenciate in medicine, a candidate had to have had a three-year apprenticeship, hold a bachelor's degree, and testify that he had no pending accounts before the Holy Office, that he had "clean blood," that he was not descended from slaves, and that he owned medical books.

The examination for the licenciate was surrounded by splendor, beginning with a mass at the cathedral at six in the morning, a parade through the streets, courtesy visits to various civic and religious authorities, and, finally, an exhaustive five-hour oral examination.

A candidate for a physician's degree, after proving he was a licenciate, was feted with a parade worthy of a king, complete with oboes, trumpets, and drums. Leading the parade were the secretary and treasurer of the university, professors of arts, medicine, and theology, and wardens and judges of the royal court; at the end came the rector, the dean of medicine, and the candidate. The ceremony for conferring the degree took place at the cathedral in the presence of the viceroy.

ROYAL COLLEGE OF SURGEONS

The eighteenth century witnessed a marked decline in medicine in Mexico; progress in learning could not keep up with that already achieved in Europe. In part this situation was due to the monopoly that Spain had over all matters in Mexico that related to culture, and the restraint the Holy Inquisition exercised over the acquirement of knowledge of new developments. Nevertheless, two positive aspects were observed: Viceroy Valero decreed that all candidates for examinations had to have had two years of practice; and the Royal College of Surgeons was founded in 1770 for the teaching of anatomy, physiology, surgery, and elements of forensic medicine. The first professorships in the college were filled by Andrés Montanéz, Manuel Antonio Moreno, Antonio Serrano y Rubio, Gutiérrez y Robledo, and Miguel García. The creation of the college was a very important development in medical-surgical studies, and the direct antecedent of the present School of Medicine.

Serious divisions became apparent, however, among medical professionals at the School of Medicine and the Royal College of Surgeons—to a certain extent they became rivals. A conflict developed between the surgeons on the faculty of the university, and the humanists at the college. The situation became worse when the college began to admit people such as barbers and bleeders, who had little formal education and for whom there were few admissions requirements, thereby increasing the competition for entrance.

Some of the published works of the eighteenth century were: *General Anthology of All Diseases* by Juan de Esteinffer; *Cursus Medicus Mexicanus* by José Salgado; *Medicinal Anthology* by Pérez Cabeza de Fierro; and *Instructions for the Curing of the Sick Afflicted with Smallpox Epidemics* by José Ignacio Bartolache, who was also the founder of the first medical review in Spanish, *El Mercurio Volante*.

PROTESTS AND REFORMS

At the beginning of the nineteenth century a protest movement prepared the way for the birth of a new university. Luis Montaña in Puebla headed this reactionary movement against doctrines governing the practice of medicine, and the decree prohibiting doctors from reading material not consistent with university policy or with the ideology of the Holy Office and Spanish politics. He fought for reforms in teaching and for more practical methods of instruction, and insisted that physics and chemistry be included in the study of medicine. "The sick give what neither corpses nor books can give," said Montaña, to emphasize the importance of practicing with patients.

The Mexican War of Independence (1810-21) marked a true transition with regard to the teaching of medicine. News of European progress in medicine—sometimes spread in a clandestine manner, sometimes openly—forced modifications to be made in existing policies, and on 2 May 1822 the Congress was forced to ask the Office of Royal Physicians to study the reforms necessitated by modern concepts of medicine and surgery. Thus the School of Medicine for the District and Territories was born.

The school eventually took over the functions of the Office of Royal Physicians, thereby ending the existence of an institution that at times was responsible for the slow development of medicine in Mexico during the colonial era. Ignorance, fanaticism, superstition, and administrative errors on the part of its members were determining factors in the backwardness of medicine in the nineteenth century, at the beginning of which the textbooks of Hippocrates and Galen had still been in use.

It is true that the Office of Royal Physicians did introduce some effective measures such as smallpox vaccination in 1797, despite the opposition, not only of the people and minor authorities but of the viceroy himself. But many of its decisions constituted a barrier to the acceptance of new ideas, methods, and criteria. An example is the defense made in 1797 by José F. Rada of bleeding as a therapeutic method, when bleeding had already been condemned by the great majority of doctors; another is the attribution of the typhus epidemic in 1813 to divine causes, according to a statement issued by the president of the Office of Royal Physicians, José García Jove, after "having thoroughly read the Sacred Scriptures."

CURRICULAR CHANGES

The School of Medicine for the District and Territories had a short life, however, and it was quickly supplanted by the Institute of Medical Sciences, whose first director, Casimiro Liceaga, had among his teaching colleagues Manuel Carpio, Pedro Escobedo, Pedro del Villar, and José Ma. Benítez.

The university's name was changed by presidential decree to the National Pontifical University. At the same time it modified its teaching crteria, and thereafter it was noted that the French pattern of instruction exerted considerable influence, especially in medicine.

After constant changes of location and many economic and other hardships—some of which were solved by the professors themselves, especially by Liceaga—in 1854 the Institute of Medical Sciences was installed in the Santo Domingo building that had been occupied by the Holy Inquisition and renamed the School of Medicine of the National

Autonomous University of Mexico. It occupied this building until 1955, when it was transferred to its present location in University City.

During the 101 years in the old building of Santo Domingo marked progress was achieved in the teaching of medicine in Mexico. One hundred generations of doctors had come out of its classrooms, leaving their footprints on the worn steps of its ancient staircase; thousands of students who passed through were lucky enough to benefit from its scientific environment. Among the illustrious figures in Mexican medicine who guided the School of Medicine during the nineteenth century were José M. Vértiz, Leopoldo Río de la Loza, Rafáel Lucio, Francisco Ortega, Manuel Carmona y Valle, and Eduardo Liceaga.

At the end of the century the medical curriculum was divided into five years: Galenic pharmacy, histology, and descriptive anatomy were studied in the first; physiology, medical pathology, surgical pathology, and clinical surgery in the second; topographic anatomy, medical and surgical pathology, and clinical medicine in the third; surgery, medical therapeutics, general pathology, and clinical surgery in the fourth; and, finally, hygiene, legal medicine, obstetrics, clinical obstetrics, and clinical medicine.

The twentieth century started with the administration of the school in the hands of Carmona y Valle. That the French concept of teaching predominated was faithfully reflected by the textbooks used: Magendie, Maygrier, Roche, Barbier, and Chevallier.

Mention should be made here of the creation, around that time, of an institute for the practical application of medicine in the battlefield. Later, during the administration of President Alvaro Obregón, this institute became the Military Medical School which today enjoys great prestige in Mexican medical circles.

During the era of the Mexican Revolution (1910-14) several personalities were responsible for the administration and direction of the School of Medicine, each of whom instituted certain teaching reforms. Among these leaders we should mention Francisco Zárraga, Rafaél Caraza, and Ulíses Valdés. The changes resulted in a greater strengthening of the curriculum and more practical activities. It was at this time, for example, that the requirement was made that students should devote a certain amount of time to laboratory and ampitheater practice. These reforms owed much to the enthusiasm, interest, and devotion shown by Rosendo Amor and Gastón Melo, among others. By 1925 the medical curriculum had been extended to six years, with a noticeable increase in the number and quality of the courses, especially microbiology, physiology, obstetrics and gynecology, pediatrics, and psychiatry.

Years later, when he successively occupied the secretariat and presidency of the school, Fernando Ocaranza instituted what he called "physiological thinking," which, in his words, consisted of "making an adequate evaluation of all dynamic facts and converting them to statistical facts."

It would be outside the scope of this brief historical synthesis to describe the events that have contributed to the structure of the medical curriculum in Mexico over the past fifty years. Suffice it to mention that during this period the teaching of medicine has been the object of multiple studies that have resulted in frequent changes in the criteria, the curriculum, and teaching methods. It is too early to assert that all modifications made during the course of these five decades have been beneficial, especially those that have been undertaken over the past twenty years.

The problems faced by professors of the stature of Ignacio Chávez, José Izquierdo, González Herrejón, Aquilino Villanueva, Gustavo Baz, and González Guzmán, to name just a few, were many and complex, but all of these people contributed to a greater or lesser extent, depending on the economic, social, and political circumstances of the times, to the advance of medicine in Mexico.

MEDICINE IN COLONIAL BRAZIL: AN OVERVIEW

Lycurgo de Castro Santos Filho

THE FIRST PHYSICIAN

Among the principal members of the expedition of Pedro Alvares Cabral to the newly discovered land of Brazil was a "Master Juan," a doctor, or "physic" as he was then called, who came to conduct astrology research and who wrote a historic letter of 1 May 1500 to King Don Manuel I of Portugal. He did not remain in Brazil, however, but continued on to India with Cabral's fleet.

Master Juan, whose name may have been Juan Faras, and whose nationality is a mystery—he could have been Spanish or German[1]—symbolized the status of medicine at that time: in addition to being a physician and an astrologer he was a cosmographer. His knowledge of medicine, however, was not enough to cure himself of "a very bad leg, that from a scratch has become a sore that is bigger than the palm of my hand," as he complained in the letter to the king.[2] Medical science, or more appropriately medical art, was still influenced by celestial bodies; was dependent on the influences of the stars; was aided by medieval alchemy; and was guided by ancient Greek and Roman principles, augmented by Arabian theories readjusted by scholastic philosophy. Empiricism governed the practice of medical art at that time.

THE LAND AND ITS DISEASES

Chroniclers who described the land of Santa Cruz, as Brazil was then called, did not stint in their praise of its salubrious climate. There were few diseases, and those who fell ill recuperated. The Indians appeared to be healthy and had sturdy constitutions. When they were ill they went to the *pajé*, witch doctor, who combined the medicinal virtues of the native flora with magic practices.

The nosographic picture at the time was relatively limited. The diseases described as most important were *bouba*, or *piã*; endemic goiters; some parasitosis and dermatosis; dysentery; unspecified fevers (rheumatism?; influenza?); respiratory disorders such as pneumonia and pleurisy; and ailments resulting from poor eating habits, poisonous reptiles, war wounds, and accidents. Many of the so-called "tropical diseases" were completely unknown in Brazil. The question of whether syphilis and malaria originated in America, or at least in Brazil, is still being debated.[3]

As colonization began, the white man's expeditions arrived, mostly from the Iberian peninsula—exploitative and commercial expeditions, coastguard contigents, pirates, and settlers. While some of the latter returned home, many remained, settled down, cohabited with Indian women, and procreated.

The white man brought his diseases with him and passed them on to the Indians, who, lacking immunizing resistance acquired through generations, fell victim to the new diseases, especially during terrible epidemics of smallpox and measles. To further enrich the pathology the white man introduced tuberculosis, scarlet fever, leprosy, parasitoses, such as a malignant itch, and other multiple ailments.

FIRST MEDICAL PROFESSIONALS

The colonizing expeditions that started in the third decade of the sixteenth century brought the first medical professionals: the "surgeon-barbers," "barbers," and "apothecaries," and their apprentices. Few in number at first, they settled in the recently founded towns along the coast, bringing with them some rudimentary principles of European science, or, more accurately, of Iberian science, for the newcomers were mostly Portuguese and Spanish. Their therapeutic arsenal consisted of instruments for surgery, bloodletting, and cutting and sawing, as well as remedies and "ingredients" (*simplices*) in their "apothecary boxes." In due course, these drugs ran out or deteriorated, however, and it became necessary to use medicinal native flora.

The individuals who practiced the medical-pharmaceutical profession during the sixteenth and seventeenth centuries were simple working men, the great majority of whom were Jews, New Christians, or semi-Christians. They were nomads whose life style was much the same as it had been in Europe; they traveled from village to village and from town to town. They would walk miles to reach a place where there was no competition, and where patients would pay for their services. They would remain there until the novelty had worn off and patients had become scarce, and then leave for another town or another farm. Some went to work for grantees, captain-generals, and farm owners; they were no more than servants in their trade.

There were some exceptions who had social status—the so-called "licensees" who had diplomas and held positions as *fisico-mors* in Salvador da Bahia, a post instituted by Tomé de Sousa, the first governor-general of Brazil. These men had letters of "authorization," enjoyed a certain amount of prestige, and received special considerations. They, too, were New Christians, who, like their colleagues, the surgeon-barbers, were accused of practicing Judaism when the first Holy Inquisition reached Brazil at the end of the sixteenth century.[4]

MIXTURE OF THE RACES

Negro slaves were first imported in 1532, and black women were soon bearing the children of white men. Thus Brazil became populated with three kinds of racial mixtures. An intense melting pot never before experienced in other regions resulted in a healthy type of individual, organically strong, well adapted to the environment, and resistent to alimentary deficiencies and adverse climatic conditions. The Brazilian, it may be said with certainty, is the result of the mixture of white, Negro, and Indian, particularly of Negro and Indian.

MORE DISEASES FOR BRAZIL

The Negro, like the white man, increased the Brazilian pathological picture with some new diseases: filariasis dracunculiasis, or "coastal bug"; yellow fever; trachoma; *máculo*;[5] ainhum, or "perforating planter disease"; goundou or paranasal exostosis; ankylostomiasis; and schistosomiasis.

JESUIT HEALERS

The Jesuits arrived in 1549 as part of the entourage of Tomé de Sousa. The priests of the Society of Jesus were to perform an important function in the development of medicine in Brazil. As in India, they devoted special care to the body in order to convert the soul. They were not only eminent missionaries, but physicians, apothecaries, and nurses. In a developing country where all resources were limited, the Jesuits took care of Indians, whites, and blacks: they provided medicine and hospitalization, performed surgery and bloodletting, and attended births. The Venerable Father José de Anchieta became famous for his care of the sick.[6]

Some of the Jesuits had studied medicine, or at least had some notion of the art; those who did not, learned it by practice. In each Jesuit college there were always brothers of the order who had received instruction during their novitiate and who acted as nurses and apothecaries. Even in the eighteenth century the only pharmacy or hospital in some villages and cities of Brazil was that attached to the Jesuit school. At the beginning their services were free, but it later became necessary to charge a modest sum for hospitalization and for prescriptions.

The Jesuits were intelligent observers who soon acquired a knowledge of Indian medicine. They identified plants with therapeutic properties and exported them to Europe, thereby adding such valuable medicinal plants as *ipecacuanha* and jaborandi to the world's pharmacopeia. Each school pharmacy kept a record in which the Jesuits copied the formulas that achieved the best results. The celebrated *Teriaca brasilica*, a typical panacea famous throughout the country, was a compound with a secret formula that was prescribed for a variety of diseases—the formula has only recently been divulged.[7]

The nosography of Brazil during the sixteenth century was developed through letters written by the Jesuits to their European correspondents. Epidemics of smallpox, measles, dysentery, and malaria, as well as other diseases that attacked the population, such as syphilis, and liver, lung, gastric, cardiac, renal, and nervous ailments, were all described in the Ignacian chronicles.

During the sixteenth and seventeenth centuries, Jesuit medicine rivaled that of the professional physicians in the art of curing, and surpassed it in terms of the Jesuits' greater efficiency, greater charity in providing treatment, and superior knowledge. The priests of Saint Ignatius undoubtedly were more knowledgeable and more cultured than the physicians and barber-surgeons who had migrated to Brazil.

DISENCHANTMENT WITH CONDITIONS

Once initial enthusiasm for the natural beauty of the country had worn off, and after the viruses that caused terrible epidemics of smallpox, measles, and yellow fever had been wiped out, there came a period of disillusionment. The stars were accused of having a malignant influence. The Europeans complained of difficulty in acclimatizing; bites of insects and poisonous reptiles; heat that produced sunstroke; high humidity; miasmic effluvia from the marshes; food that was difficult to digest; and the excessively savage nature of conditions in general. They cursed the tropical climate and the native diseases that constantly endangered their health. Such criticisms were voiced by chroniclers and voyagers who went back to Europe, and Brazil reached the nineteenth century with a reputation for its deplorable climatic and sanitary conditions.

THE HOLY HOUSES OF MERCY

The need to hospitalize indigent patients and recent arrivals with neither family nor homes brought about the creation of "Santa Casas," "Holy Houses of Mercy" similar to those founded in Lisbon in 1498. The first was probably the house organized by Brás Cubas in 1543 in the port of Santos;[8] others were later founded in the principal cities and towns. Together with the Jesuit infirmaries, these houses aided the indigent sick and the rich alike during epidemics. Other hospitals included that maintained for the army, which was operated by the government; public quarantine wards for lepers and victims of medical deformities; and isolation wards for carriers of contagious diseases. Lack of operating funds, a scarcity of medicines, and poor technical competence plagued the hospitals of the colonial era, however: a hospital was more than a depository for the sick; it was an antechamber to death.

THE MEDICAL PROFESSIONALS

Professionals who practiced medicine in Brazil up to the beginning of the nineteenth century were called physicians or licensees, surgeon-barbers, approved surgeons, or examined surgeons. Those who had received their diplomas from a European school, usually Portuguese or Spanish, occupied posts as physicians to the crown, the senate of the chamber, and the army. They lived in the principal cities and villages, were few in number, and their medical knowledge was not extensive, because, according to a chronicler of the nineteenth century, "physicians who possess a knowledge of science and a character are generally the last to settle in a relatively new country."

The surgeon-barbers therefore comprised the greater part of the medical profession. Their practice was limited to surgery, after they had taken an examination before, and had been approved by, the health authorities. In fact, however, because of the shortage of physicians, the surgeon-barbers practiced all branches of medicine. They, too, lived in the cities and towns, and many of them held positions with the army, the senate, and other sectors of the administration. But the surgeon-barbers had even less knowledge of medicine than the physicians, and the barbers were their greatest competitors. The barbers had no formal education and were of a low social class; some were freed slaves. They were also required to take an examination in bloodletting, cutting, the application of cupping glasses, and the extraction of teeth. They were to be found in villages, towns, and cities, where they tried to pass as physicians whenever possible.

As capable professionals were few and the territorial expansion vast, others who practiced medicine included apothecaries and their apprentices; apprentices to barbers and surgeon-barbers; *anatomicos*; *algebristas*; and other quacks.

The practice of medicine was not very lucrative for these itinerant professionals. It was not until the middle of the seventeenth century that

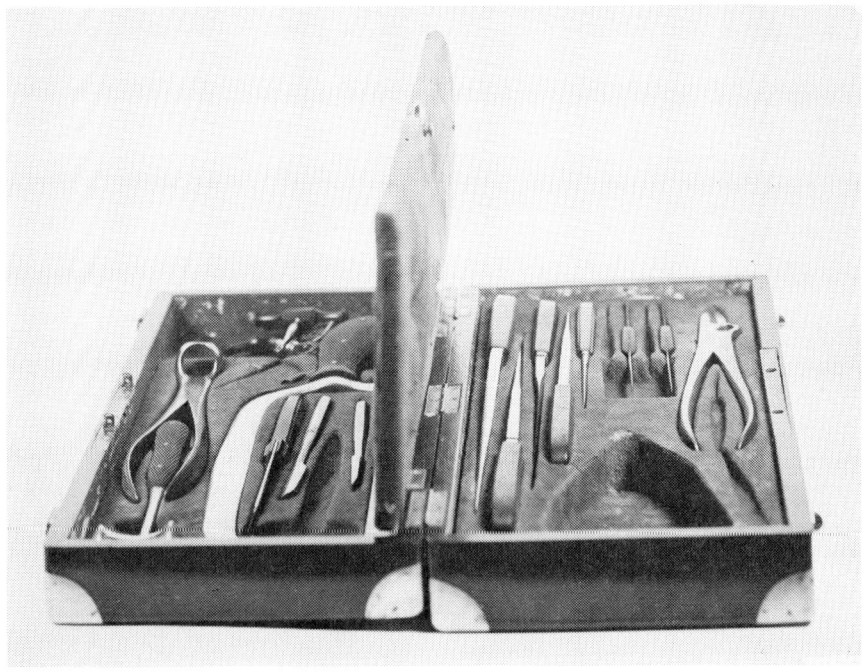

Contents of surgeon's case. Property of José Manuel de Castro Santos (1822-74) who practiced in the city of Guaratingueta, São Paulo Province, Brazil. He was the great-great-grandfather of the author.

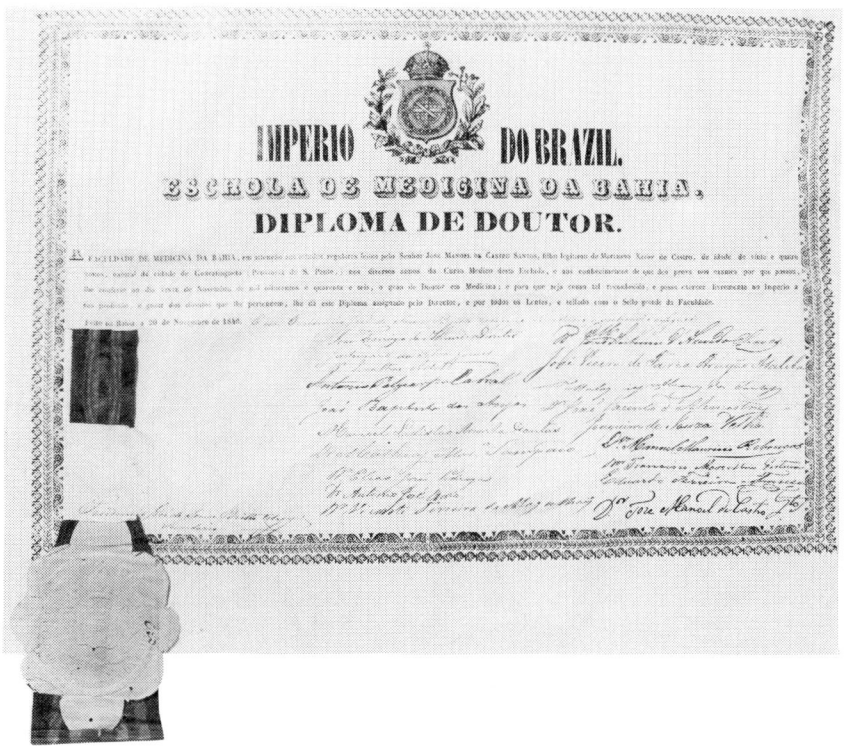

Medical diploma awarded in 1846 to José Manuel de Castro Santos from the School of Medicine of Bahia. Founded in 1808, the school was the first in Brazil.

licensed physicians were able to move up the social ladder and become integrated with the middle classes in the cities. Economic conditions gradually improved, however, as did the cultural level of the practitioners. The first known Brazilian medical bibliography was produced in the seventeenth century.

ADMINISTRATION

Supervision of professional practice and the sale of drugs fell under the jurisdiction of delegates or officers of the first exchequer and the chief surgeon of the kingdom until 1782, when the government of Maria I of

Portugal created the Board of the First Medical House, which was located in Lisbon with representatives in Brazil. They gave examinations to candidates (*cartas de examinação*) to practice as surgeon-barbers and barbers; cancelled diplomas and licenses; inspected pharmacies; established the prices of drugs; visited hospitals; issued sanitation measures during times of epidemics; and supervised the practices of physicians, surgeon-barbers, barbers, and midwives. They were governed by regulations and authorizations that were issued periodically.

SANITARY MEASURES

As there were few sanitary officials, their activities were varied. When epidemics broke out, proclamations from the captain-generals regulated matters concerning hygiene and health, and determined such activities as street and house cleanings, isolation of patients, closing of ports, and prescriptions for preventive medicines; they imprisoned those who disobeyed the decrees.

The senates of the chambers of the villages and cities also regulated hygiene measures and, through their "party" doctors, watched over the health of the people by supervising the medical and pharmaceutical professions within the limits of the scant funds available.

SCIENTIFIC RESEARCH

The first 300 years of Brazilian medicine produced no doctors who undertook research, made any scientific observations worthy of mention, or stood out in a specialized branch, such as sanitation measures. The environment was not appropriate. Some physicians did gain reputations for their superior knowledge or for their skill and subtlety in the practice of their profession. Some were devoted to the study of botany; others studied and recorded endemic and epidemic diseases. Their published works retain a special place in the Brazilian medical bibliography.

DUTCH MEDICINE

The occupation of north and northeast Brazil by the Dutch during the seventeenth century brought medical professionals of various nationalities, almost all of them Jewish, to the territories under Dutch domain.

most important medical professionals integrated the social literature of the Scientific Academy and the Literary Society, both in Rio. One of them, Manuel Joaquim Henriques de Paiva, who was later to gain importance as a physician in Lisbon, published numerous books. At the time of his death in Bahia he was a professor at the Medical-Surgical Academy.

No periodicals or reviews of a medical or pharmaceutical nature existed at that time.

CLINICAL SCHOOL

To the general panorama outlined here we should add that medicine in colonial Brazil was not oriented toward the theories or principles then proclaimed. Nevertheless, if we were to describe medicine as it was practiced it could very well be a "clinical" school of observation of symptoms at the patient's bedside. It was of course an individualized and isolated school, with no pupils, that disappeared with its professor, who was unable to transmit his system of perspicacity and intuition in clinical interpretation.

NOTES

1. Frazão Vasconcelos, "Um documento inédito que importa à história de marinharia dos descobrimentos," *Separate de Petrus Nonius* (Lisboa) 1 (1937).
2. *História da Expansão Portuguesa no Mundo*, 3 vols. (Lisbon: Editorial Atica, 1937-40). Transcription and interpretation of the letter from Master Juan.
3. Pathology became known through the writings of the chroniclers and the first settlers, and especially through the Jesuits' letters. There is no proof that syphilis and malaria existed in Brazil at the time of the discovery; these diseases came after colonization.
4. The first visit of the Holy Inquisition to Brazil occurred when Portugal became a Spanish domain during the time of the Philips. It resulted in precious documents that are deposited in the archives of the Torre del Tombo in Lisbon. Published under the sponsorship of a wealthy São Paulo intellectual, Paulo Prado, the work offered varied and invaluable reports on social and economic life in the sixteenth century. When writing the *History of Medicine in Brazil from the Sixteenth to the Nineteenth Centuries*, 2 vols. (São Paulo: Editoria Brasiliense, 1947), the author made use of that valuable material.
5. The diseases brought by the Negroes were described by chroniclers and medical writers. The *máculo*, or *doença do bicho*, or even the *corrupção*, was described by all writers as a strange ailment. The treatment was extremely painful, consisting of introducing *sacatrapos* or *bolos de massa forte* (a mixture of lemon juice, tobacco, pepper, alcohol, and gunpowder) into the anus of a patient, who stood on his head close to a wall. Miguel Dias Pimenta wrote one of the first books about the disease in Brazilian medical literature: *Noticias do que e o achaque do Bicho* (Lisbon: n.p., 1707). More modern tropicalists, however, confessing ignorance of its true etiology, have classified the *máculo* as "gangrenous rectitis." Eustaquio Duarte, in *Morão, Rosa and Pimenta, Noticia sobre los tres primeros libros de Medicina escritos en el Brasil* (Recife: State Public

Archives, 1956), calls it ulcerating rectitis following dysentery and complications by the miasis...."—parasites in the larvae of flies.

      6. From the time of their arrival in 1549 until their expulsion by order of the Marquis de Pombal in 1759, the Jesuits converted, taught second-grade pupils in their schools, and provided hospital, medical, and pharmaceutical services. The Jesuit letters and other periodic reports to their superiors are other sources of documentary information on the history of Indian, Negro, and Iberian medicine. Father José de Anchieta became the symbol of the missionary doctor. During his life in Brazil he was a physician, surgeon-barber, nurse, midwife, and apothecary. In the *Anchietana* (São Paulo: National Commission for the Commemoration of Anchieta's Day, 1965), the present author proclaimed this Jesuit to be the foremost medical figure in sixteenth century Brazil.

      7. In his book, *Arts an Works of the Jesuits in Brazil (1549-1760)* (Lisbon and Rio de Janeiro: Ediciones Broteira, Libro de Portugal, 1953), Father Serafin Leite quoted from the manuscript, "Coleção de Receitas do Arquivo Romano da Companhia de Jesus," a series of sixty-two "specific" compositions prepared by the Jesuits in Brazil, and even the formula for *Teriaca brasilica*—a mixture of extracts from the roots of native and foreign plants, oils, rubbers, and mineral salts—which was a panacea for the symptoms of all known diseases.

      8. There is a scarcity of documents describing the first Brazilian Holy Houses of Mercy. The minutes of their meetings were burned by Dutch, English, and French invaders and pirates. The holy houses of Santos, Salvador da Bahia, and Olinda in Pernambuco, are said by historians to have been the first, but the actual dates of their foundation are not known. The hospitals of mercy, fashioned after the one in Lisbon that was sponsored and protected by the Queen Dowager Doña Leonor of Portugal, were worthy charitable institutions the Portuguese brought to the lands they discovered.

      9. The second book written by Simão Pinhēiro Morão, *Queixas repetidas em ecos dos arrecifes de Pernambuco contra os abusos medicos que nas capitanias se observam tanto en dano das vidas seus habitantes* (Lisbon: Junta de Investigaciones de Ultramar, 1965) is available today.

     10. João Ferreira da Rosa, *Tratado único da constituição pestilencial de Pernambuco* (Lisbon: n.p., 1694). This work on yellow fever seems to have been the first in specialized international literature to deal with this disease.

     11. Dias Pimenta, *Noticias do Bicho* (See note 5).

DISCUSSANT:

Donald B. Cooper

Lycurgo de Castro Santos Filho's concise and scholarly panorama of the medical history of colonial Brazil offers an excellent introduction to an important though somewhat neglected field of study. As all historians of medicine in Latin America know, Santos Filho has for many years made a determined effort to expand our knowledge of this subject. His two-volume work, *História da medicina no Brasil*,[1] remains our best general account of Brazilian colonial medicine, and his *Pequena história da medicina Brasileira* provides many new details, particularly of the postcolonial period.[2]

     One still has the feeling, however, that much more is known about the medical histories of New Spain and colonial Peru, and possibly of the Maya and the Incas, than that of Brazil from 1500 to 1822. One obvious reason for this neglect is the relative scarcity of sources. Brazil had no printing press until the arrival of Dom João Sexto in 1808. While several works on medicine, including a few of outstanding importance, were published in Portugal during the colonial period, Brazil had neither newspapers nor journals, and the items printed in Portugal were fewer in number than those printed in either Mexico or Peru during the same period. Furthermore, there has been a severe loss of manuscript sources. A great many certainly were lost during the Lisbon earthquake and tidal wave of 1 November 1755, which destroyed a large part of the Portuguese archives.

Another reason for the relative neglect of Brazilian colonial medical history is than in the medical area, as in the political and economic areas, the course of events in Brazil was much less dramatic than in Spanish America. Politically the colony produced no great and systematic plunder of rich and sophisticated Indian societies, such as happened in Mexico, Peru, and Colombia in the sixteenth century. Economically Brazil lived for nearly two centuries on the lucrative but unspectacular resources of her forests and fields, while her settlers hugged the coastline almost within sight of the Atlantic ocean. It was a colony whose urban centers were for the most part mere gathering points for the distribution of the fruits of the land.

Similarly, in the medical field one finds fewer widespread epidemics than in New Spain and the Caribbean. As Santos Filho states, while Brazil did suffer from severe outbreaks of smallpox and malaria, they were evidently not comparable to the great pandemic of smallpox that struck Middle America and Peru between 1514 and 1530, or to the deadly epidemics of yellow fever in the Caribbean and in Mexico in the seventeenth and eighteenth centuries. This may have meant a more pleasant and healthful existence for residents of Brazil, but it also may have caused historians, particularly foreign historians, to overlook the country's rich tapestry of medical history.

Santos Filho's paper suggests several very fruitful areas of investigation that might be worthy starting points for in-depth studies. Serafim Leite is said to have stated that one cannot write seriously about Brazilian colonial history without taking into account the extraordinary role of the Jesuits. For 210 years (1549-1759) they were centrally involved in Brazil's religious, political, social, and economic affairs, and, as Santos Filho makes clear, their role in medicine was no less important. The good fathers labored to save the bodies as well as the souls of their charges, be they white, red, or black. José de Anchieta, Manoel da Nobrega, and Antonio de Vieira set an example in their concern for the sick and the poor, and they were emulated by hundreds of lesser-known men of this remarkable order, many of whom were martyred en route to and while in Brazil. Yet it seems fair to say that we still lack a full and completely objective study of the Jesuit influence on Brazilian medicine.

Without questioning the good intentions of the followers of Saint Ignatius, however, one wonders to what extent the Jesuits themselves were responsible for introducing new and deadly diseases into Indian communities. The Jesuits were, after all, frequently the advance agents of the crown, the persons who initiated and maintained contact between the Indians and the Portuguese. Did the insistence of the order that Indians be coerced into urban communities so they might be more effectively catechized and put to work make these primitive people "sitting ducks" for contagious diseases? To what extent was medical care available to Indians who had not been catechized or baptized? And, finally, why did the Jesuits study and accept so much Indian lore on drugs and medicines while rejecting, even castigating, so many other features of traditional Indian society? There should be plentiful material for a fuller study of Jesuit influence in medicine, even though most of the sources were written by Jesuits.

Another interesting but lesser topic relating medicine and religion is the medical role of Jews and New Christians in colonial Brazil. Considering the more tolerant nature of the Portuguese, and the absence in Brazil of the dread Inquisition, it was in fact possible for Jews and New Christians to participate more or less openly in Brazilian society. Santos Filho makes it very clear that they were important at virtually all levels of medical practice, from humble pharmacists, to wandering *curandeiros*, to graduated and licensed physicians. Such an assertion seems less than surprising when one remembers that from the earliest days New Christians were important in Brazil; Fernando de Noronha, the explorer and entrepreneur, was a member of this group.

Yet I must admit to some slight skepticism regarding the veracity of contemporary accounts of the numbers and influence of Jews and New Christians. Dutch businessmen in Recife in 1641 claimed that "all the Jews in the world are moving here"—a slight exaggeration to be sure; nor were the Spanish correct in their oft-repeated assertion that virtually every Portuguese merchant, trader, or *peruleiro* who entered their domain was a New Christian or a Jew. Possibly it is true that virtually all Dutch physicians were of Jewish descent, as Santos Filho suggests, yet the Calvinists seem to have complained as much as the Portuguese about the New Christians of Pernambuco. In any event there is no doubt that Jews and New Christians played a major role in Brazilian colonial medicine, and only a minor one in Spanish colonial medicine.

Neither the Jesuits nor the New Christians contributed any sizeable number of licensed and graduated physicians. The medical regulars were all trained in Europe, mainly at Coimbra, since the Portuguese crown repeatedly refused to meet the colony's demands for a university. There seems no reason at all to question Santos Filho's assertion that such men were relatively few in number, that they often preferred to treat wealthy *fazendeiros*, members of the armed forces, and city dwellers, and that most of them were, and have remained, relatively obscure figures. As far as we know, none carried out any medical research or experimentation worthy of mention, unless we include works based on keen powers of observation, such as João Ferriera da Rosa's classic description of yellow fever.[3]

In closing I would say that Santos Filho does a masterful job of identifying the leading themes and problems of Brazilian colonial medical history. Future investigators will no doubt seek to expand the horizons of our somewhat limited knowledge in this field. Records are sparse and many important questions and controversies are yet to be settled. It would be very helpful if a complete bibliography were to be prepared, bringing together all the widely scattered manuscripts and printed sources on Brazilian colonial medical history. But even were this available it is likely that any historian attempting to become oriented in this field would turn, as I once did, to the works of the historian, Lycurgo de Castro Santos Filho, whose *História da Medicina no Brasil* remains the single most valuable account available.

NOTES

1. Lycurgo Santos Filho, *História da medicina no Brasil (Do século XVI ao século XIX)*, 2 vols. (São Paulo: Editoria Brasiliense, 1947; Coleção "Grandes Estudos Brasilienses," vols. III and IIIA).

2. _____, *Pequena história da medicina Brasileira* (São Paulo: São Paulo Editoria, 1966; Coleção Buruti).

3. João Ferreira da Rosa, *Tratado único da constituição pestilencial de Pernambuco* (Lisbon:n.p., 1694).

THE TEACHING OF MEDICINE IN COLONIAL COLOMBIA

A. Seriano Lleras

The teaching of medicine was introduced to New Granada, part of which is now Colombia, by Francisco Díaz, a Spanish physician who practiced in Santa Fé de Bogotá. Díaz instructed a local man, Juan López, in the science of medicine and eventually took him to Salamanca, where he graduated. López returned to Santa Fé in 1584.

No further effort to teach medicine was made until March 1636, when Licenciado Rodrigo Enríquez de Andrade, a Spanish physician who had graduated from Alcalá, came to New Granada. He had been given the title of chief physician (*protomédicus*) by the president of the colony, the Marquis of Sofraga. Upon his arrival he requested a readership in medicine from the Royal Court of Spain as follows:

> Very powerful Sir. I, Licenciado Rodrigo Enríquez de Andrade, have had notice that there are in this city professorships of Arts and Teutology, but there is an absence, for the adornment of this Court, of someone to read the Medicine course, [and] to be able to create physicians without having to send to Spain for them; also, that there are many who are inclined to this profession but have not studied because of the lack of teaching, nor do they practice their abilities. . . . from your lordship I request authorization so that I may read this course on Medicine in whichever part you see fit, for it is great honor and to the advantage of all this Court that I be so appointed. *Licenciado Enríquez.*

This was a more advanced step than that taken by Díaz, as Enríquez wanted to open the study of medicine to anyone inclined toward it who was qualified to take the course. At the same time, the move was a way of fighting against taxation, which seems to have been onerous.

The memorandum to the Royal Court was received favorably, and the request was granted "without this implying the acquisition of any rights, nor that the hearers shall approve any courses." At the same time, the court asked the rector of the university, a Jesuit, to choose the most appropriate classroom in which to teach the course.

The same room used for the philosophy course was chosen, and the time for the reading of medicine was fixed at 8:15 in the morning. Enríquez inaugurated his instructions in Latin, in accordance with the practice of the rector and other Jesuit teachers and of the many religious and lay pupils. The course began on 1 April 1636.

Two years later Enríquez requested permission to request some tuition fees from the students "because it somehow seems indecent that being a member of this university, I should only be entitled to read the course and not to receive the same income as the other professors receive for their work." In exchange for such remuneration, he offered to become the private physician to the faculty of the university.

The Assembly of the senior members of the university, according to minutes of their subsequent meetings,

> decided for very serious reasons, that the said professor, Don Rodrigo, should not be admitted to the faculty, but should only be the professor of medicine in this school, with the approval of the Royal Court. As Chief Physician he would be the doctor in charge of giving treatment to doctors and teachers of the said Academy, and for this service he should receive the same fee as a teacher, both from the present students as well as from those who have graduated; that he should not wear a tassel for these purposes, but only a short cape; and if he should break this agreement, a fine will be levied to him, the amount to be left to the judgment of the Rector, and the decision made by him.

Enríquez was not satisfied with this resolution and complained that "a terrible affront was being done to him, with detriment to the academy itself, in as much as he was a professor of the academy." Thereupon "the university withdrew its resolution in view of the fact that Enríquez was a dean of the school and its founder and first professor of medicine, and he was allowed to wear a tassel and to receive fees on the same basis as the other professors."

As chief physician, Enríquez examined all medical candidates and granted licenses to practice the profession. By 1641 the medical course was no longer being given due to a lack of students, and Enríquez was therefore deprived of an income, a measure he protested against saying that he should continue to receive what little money was given him because he had been publicly awarded the title of professor "to read for a small remuneration; otherwise a legal statement be made stating that I am not a professor and orders be given to attest this matter."

Father Mas, the rector, ordered that this complaint be referred to the students so they could state their opinion on the matter, and a decision could be taken. Enríquez insisted on his rights and, furthermore, requested that the students deposit with the university the fees owed to him until the issue was definitely settled. This request was accepted.

On 31 December 1651, Philip IV signed a royal decree by which he "gave authorization to the Archbishop of Santa Fé de Bogotá to establish a school for the study of the doctrines of Saint Thomas, Law and Medicine." Juan Francisco Párano, "the only one with the necessary attributes" became rector of the new school.

In 1653 Fray Cristóbal de Torres requested authorization from the Cabinet of Madrid to establish the Superior College of Our Lady of the Rosary. The school was to have a professorship in beginning medicine, but it could not be established at the time because there was no qualified person to take it.

A royal decree of 20 September 1673 ordered the Chapter of Santa Fé to "adjudge the necessary funds to keep the Professor of Medicine at the Superior College of Our Lady of the Rosary." Another decree in the same year, issued in the name of the queen and addressed to the Royal Court and the Chapter of Santa Fé, requested that the necessary steps be taken to provide funds to create the professorship of medicine, and that the sovereign be informed of the results.

José de la Cruz was graduated from the School of the Superior College of Our Lady of the Rosary in 1715, and the chapter appointed him as chief physician and professor of beginning medicine at the school, but he did not accept the professorship.

Francisco de Fuentes, a medical graduate of Palermo, arrived in Santa Fé in 1732. His title as physician was confirmed on 1 February 1733, and he was requested to take over the professorship of medicine, "with a donation from the Chapter," at the Superior College of Our Lady of the Rosary. The appointment was dated 16 September 1733 and signed by Rafaél de Eslaba y Caballero, governor and captain general of New Granada.

Fuentes assumed the professorship on 23 October, but no students registered for the course as a medical career was considered demeaning, fit only for people of very low social status. There was, nevertheless, an inaugural class attended by five scholars, two university students, and two friars, one a physician from the religious order of San Juan de Dios. In 1734 Fuentes left the city and went to Caracas where he took up residence.

Years later there was a move to revive the professorship of medicine. Vicente Román Cancino was considered to be a candidate for the post, but he was unable to accept it because he lacked a degree. He took an examination at the University of Saint Thomas, however, and graduated in October 1753. The then rector, Nicolás de Vargas, appointed Cancino professor of medicine, and he conducted his classes without order, method, or regularity until his death in 1766.

In 1758 there was an attempt to replace Cancino with Juan José Courtois, who was granted the appointment but did not accept it because he had been so long in medical practice he had forgotten the theory of medical science. He later became a professor at the University of Saint Thomas. In the course of his stay in Santa Fé he changed his name to Cortés.

José Celestino Mutis, a physician from Cadiz, arrived in Cartagena on 29 October 1760. He had completed four theoretical courses in medicine at Seville: beginning medicine, prelude to medicine, anatomy, and surgery. When he had completed those courses he returned to Cadiz, where he entered the obligatory two years of practice under the direction of Pedro Fernández de Castilla, going to the Marine Hospital daily and attending all dissections conducted, as well as participating in other scientific activities in the hospital. Mutis returned to Seville, where he graduated as a bachelor of medicine in May 1755. He returned to practice for a short time in Cadiz and then went to Madrid, where he took an examination and was awarded the doctoral degree in July 1757. He was appointed assistant professor of anatomy at the university under Doctor Aráujo.

From a medical point of view the arrival of Mutis in New Granada was very important, as he was an extremely well-qualified individual who was to give great impetus to the medical profession, especially with regard to teaching.

In 1761 Miguel de Isla entered the San Juan de Díos Hospital, where he began his practical studies in medicine under the guidance of Fray Antonio de Guzmán. Isla, with Mutis, was later to play an important role in teaching.

When Cancino graduated Juan Bautista de Vargas Uribe in January 1764, Mutis attended the ceremony. Vargas was the only student graduated by Cancino.

Upon Cancino's death in 1766 the professorship of medicine was offered to Mutis, who was by then the personal physician of the viceroy, Messía de la Zerda. The Royal Court requested the appointment from the crown, which asked the opinion of the viceroy, who answered by saying that with the appointment of Mutis we will have capable physicians in this city, which up to now has had only those who come from the outside, and has been forced to rely on them without stopping to verify their abilities or the legitimacy of their titles.

Mutis refused the appointment, however, because he preferred to devote his time to scientific investigations.

The rector of the Superior College of Our Lady of the Rosary, Miguel de Masustegui, thereupon called for a competitive examination to be given. Vargas took the tests, which were given by laymen such as the lawyers Antonio González Manrique and Manuel de Rubiales. Mutis and a surgeon, Jaime Navarro, attended as guests.

Another disciple of Cancino was Juan José Cortés, who had been established for some time in Tunja when the viceroy appointed him as chief physician of Santa Fé, without the obligation of taking over the professorship of medicine. But the license was denied by the Chapter of Santa Fé after a long dispute, because Vargas asked the mayoralty to annul the appointment of Cortés and to grant it to him.

To obtain the post of chief physician that had been denied him by the chapter, Cortés

> was graduated as a doctor from the University of Saint Thomas. He offered [Doctor Masustegui] ... to take over the Professorship of Medicine on condition that he be exempted from the obligatory competitive tests. This request was denied by the rector as "it was not within his jurisdiction to grant this grace."

Vargas's request that Cortés's appointment be annulled was based on the fact that he already had an appointment as professor of medicine at the Superior College of Our Lady of the Rosary with the approval of the viceroy, and that the two posts could not be held by the same man. Cortés intervened by submitting certificates of good management from his medical colleagues in Santa Fé, who, besides Vargas, were Guzmán, Navarro, and José de Atriesta. Furthermore, he presented a certificate from the rector "that proved he had requested the professorship of medicine without taking competitive tests."

Asked for their opinion on the matter, Mutis and Navarro both favored Cortés, who, supported by existing laws, asked that Vargas be debarred from the profession. Vargas protested, presenting the legal credentials granted by Cancino and many certificates by rich and influential people attesting that he practiced medicine effectively.

> At the beginning of 1766 the Royal Court confirmed the appointment of Doctor Cortés as Chief Physician, exempting him from the obligation of taking

over the Professorship, a disposition which was contrary to the order of that Court of July 21, 1760. In January 1767 the viceroy appointed Vargas as the professor of beginning medicine. The possibility of resolving the dispute increased, however, when Cortés suddenly left the city, and subsequently abandoned New Granada by the end of 1767.

During his tenure at the Superior College, Cortés granted licences to Atriesta and Diego Crespo, but denied a licence to Henbamberg, a Danish physician, even though the Chapter of Santa Fé had granted the latter a licence because he was newly converted to Catholicism. Cortés also granted licences to Manuel Ignacio, Antonio Froes, and Alejandro Gastelbondo, and to the apothecaries Antonio Garroes and Fray José Bohorquez, a friar of the Order of San Juan de Dios.

In 1768 Vargas inaugurated the course on introduction to medicine and gave some lectures on the circulation of the blood, but because of his lack of scientific knowledge he was forced to relinquish the professorship. Subsequently he left the city.

The Royal Court of Santa Fé, aware of the superior medical knowledge of Mutis, requested the king to grant him the title of chief physician on condition that he not return to Spain until he had trained capable disciples who could replace him. The viceroy advised the king that he had engaged Mutis as his personal physician because of his great confidence in Mutis's skills.

Vargas returned to Santa Fé in 1773 hoping to establish the beginning medicine course, but Attorney General Francisco Moreno y Escandón had drawn up teaching reforms that were to be initiated in 1774. There was thus to be no opportunity for Vargas to continue teaching as he had before. He then took an examination at Angelica University, and in its registrar is an entry attesting that, on 17 January 1774, Vargas was graduated and the medical degree conferred on him. The certificate is signed by Fray Luis Nieves, as rector, and Fray Jacinto Buenaventura, Antonio Manrique, and Manuel Rubieles, as professors, although they probably knew less about the medical sciences than the graduate himself, who at least had been an apothecary.

Vargas conducted the beginning medicine course until 1774, when, because of the implementation of the new curriculum, orders were given to discontinue classes at the college until further notice. In this short tenure Vargas did not train any disciples.

In the following year Viceroy Caballero y Góngora drew up a new study plan and proposed the creation of two courses, beginning medicine and a prelude to medicine, at a new university. The courses were to be given by two Spanish physicians and were to be patterned after the programs of the best schools of the Iberian peninsula; but this concept did not become a reality.

In 1777 Isla offered to read the medicine course, but as there was no chief physician in Santa Fé, he had no legal authority to teach or to practice and he therefore returned to Cali.

The rector of the Superior College of Our Lady of the Rosary next offered the professorship of medicine to Sebastián López Ruíz, a Panamanian doctor who had graduated from the University of San Marcos in Lima, where he had been a professor. López did not accept the appointment, however, because it offered no remuneration.

Mutis administered the medicine course from 1774 to 1778, but in a very haphazard manner, and his teaching was not well regarded by some people in Santa Fé. The course was eliminated in 1778 by the Superior Board of Education, which was created by royal decree on 18 July of that year.

The study plan of the new medical professorship was drawn up by Viceroy Guairior and the Superior Board of Admissions, which was integrated by the viceroy and the diocesan prelate, José Gregorio Díaz Quijano; the dean of the judges of the court, José Joaquín de Aróstegui y Escoto; José Antonio Peñalver, the attorney general of the king; and Francisco Moreno y Escandón, the protector of the Indians. The professorship was reestablished in Santa Fé in 1784, with the course being conducted by Francisco Vergara.

As there had been no professor of medicine at the Superior College of Our Lady of the Rosary since 1768, Isla offered to take on the task without reimbursement, but the head priest of the Jesuit order begged the viceroy not to allow this because he thought it would harm the order.

In 1793 the Secular Chapter of Popayán requested permission from the Royal Court to create three courses in medicine at the Seminary College, but Charles IV refused to grant authorization.

The rector of the Superior College of Our Lady of the Rosary, Fernando Caycedo y Flórez, wanted to establish a professorship of medicine in the capital so that the educational plan approved by the college would be on firm ground. He therefore requested the viceroy to institute a complete educational policy, adding that, in his opinion, Mutis was the most appropriate person to direct it as he knew the subject very well and was also aware of the economic limitations of the college because he had once been the mathematics professor there.

Isla still wanted to graduate as a doctor of medicine, but there was no way he could take the prescribed course. He therefore asked the court to dispense with the legal formalities and award him the title. But the attorney general compelled the priest to take a public examination given by Mutis. In March 1798 Mutis advised the viceroy that he was ready to verify the revalidation examination of Isla, as requested, so that he could teach medicine. After praising Isla highly, Mutis said that

> although there may be many professors to choose from, no one surpasses Professor Isla in the performance of his duties in the professorship. His abilities, his involvement in all natural sciences, his constant application, his genius for teaching (of which he has given proof in private courses)—of all this I am well assured by his last examination. He answered with great dignity all the questions I deemed essential in order to issue this report in compliance with my mission. This aspiring doctor has the title of military physician with authority to choose hospital patients for the instruction of students in the clinic. You will therefore be aware of the great opportunity presented to Your Excellency for such a worthy professor to begin teaching for the benefit of all the provinces of the viceroyship that are exposed to ignorant quacks and foreign charlatans who are tolerated by the Government because of the lack of qualified doctors.

Despite such testimony the attorney general was still opposed to Isla taking over the professorship.

On 2 April 1799 Rector Caycedo again requested the king to establish the professorship of medicine. On 7 June Viceroy Mendinueta decided that, since Isla had been qualified as a doctor, he could temporarily take over the professorship, and that Mutis should present for his study and approval a plan for the School of Medicine.

In view of these developments, the rector presented a memorandum to the viceroy. In it he explained that, because of the death of Vargas twenty-six years before, the professorship of medicine had been discontinued, despite the fact that the viceroyship had been requesting it; the rectors of the college, the Chapter of Santa Fé, the Royal Court, and the government had exhausted their efforts to revive the professorship. In conclusion the rector wrote:

> Just when we had hoped to see in a short time many able young men in this capital devoted to the glorious study of such a necessary field for humanity, in courses methodically conducted by an able and modest professor, who would have the best textbooks as a guide, in accordance with the plan I requested, Your Excellency, in his decree of June 7, 1799 ordered that it be integrated by Doctor Mutis, who of course would be one of the best people. Just when we hoped that all of this would come about, new difficulties and obstacles have appeared that are delaying the implementation of the courses.
>
> The inauguration of all of the courses requires, My Lord, (in the opinion

of this Rector, who respectfully requests it), that Your Excellency increase your reports to the King, Our Lord, so that His Majesty, by an order from his sovereign authority, will not only untangle but stop the new complications that hinder the reestablishment of such an important professorship at once.

What a comfort it would be for all the sick people of this Kingdom if they could know that Medicine is being taught with careful attention and consistency. With what confidence they could place themselves in the hands of a physician who had studied and practiced according to true principles, so they could conceive a well-founded hope of recovering their health? And not (as happens many times) to have to place themselves in the hands of quacks and foreigners, who, after being consulted and obeyed because of the need, suddenly disappear because they do not want to take the responsibility for the ravages they cause, of which many dismal examples can be given.

It is through these means (as we hope from the pity of Our Sovereign) that the clamor from so many worthy citizens will be silenced, for they have been requesting and begging for such a long time for the establishment of this professorship, as true lovers of humanity. A privilege will then have been restored to my college which it has been deprived of for so many years. Your Excellency himself will see the benefits that you have always stated you desire for the good of this kingdom you guide so well. The honorable name of our King will be pronounced and repeated with thousands of blessings and praises by so many sick people who will owe their relief, their comfort, and perhaps the complete recovery of their health to the generous hand of the sovereign who, as a Universal Father of these loyal subjects, untangled with one blow all the knots and all obstacles that up to now have hindered the realization of our desires.

This is all with regard to the matter that I can and must inform Your Excellency with.

Superior College of Our Lady of the Rosary of Santa Fé. Excellency. Lord.

Fernando Caicedo

Despite this entreaty, Attorney General Blaya ordered that classrooms were not to be opened until the court approved the resolution of the viceroy. The rector then requested the intervention of the chapter, because it had the obligation and the right to take action on problems related to public health; the matter was therefore transferred to the court.

On 19 July 1800 the viceroy addressed the court, saying that Isla had requested exemption from the legal requirements necessary to receive a doctor's degree, and that Attorney General Blaya was opposed to this; and that Isla had then been told he must take an examination before Mutis, who considered him very competent to teach the course, which was so necessary. The viceroy then requested that the king grant the necessary authorization to Isla.

A royal decree of 28 September 1801 ordered the separation of the schools of medicine and surgery, and decreed that these professorships were to be considered independent of each other, but with equal standing.

By royal decree, Isla was appointed as professor of medicine on 2 October 1802; Mutis was appointed regent of studies; and Don Vicente Gil de Tejada was appointed assistant professor. Isla's appointment was temporary, however, and took into account the opinions of the Council of Indies and of the attorney general of the kingdom. The decree added:

> And as it is agreeable that this professorship be fully endowed, I have resolved that, through a Hearing of the Rector and the Assembly of the University, the Rector of the College of the Rosary, and the Civil Attorney General, you begin to keep a record as soon as possible, if you are not able through the funds and means of the University to meet the endowment of said professorship that you deem so necessary, you may call on the surplus funds of that Capital, and, if there are none, to the provinces of the kingdom that have them; in the absence of all of them, you should then propose to me the tax that is the least onerous to the public, that I might consider applicable, after hearing the consultative vote of this my Royal Court. That whilst the circumstances of that kingdom are improved, and whilst we obtain the reaction of the Physicians of the Court according to the laws, as in other capitals of my domains, to watch over the conduct of the professors, to examine and approve those who have the necessary abilities to be entrusted with the preservation of public health; that the mentioned Director of the Botanical Expedition, don José Mutis, Professor of Medicine, don Miguel de Isla, and another physician of that city whom you might consider fit and proper, take care of the necessary examinations so there might be three examiners in number as in these my kingdoms, giving an account of everything for my Royal approval.

The viceroy ordered the opening of the medical courses with a plan of study identical to that of the Spanish schools. The plan was presented to the government in October 1802, was approved, and was put into effect in December.

The importance of the teaching of mathematics and the natural sciences was made evident in the curriculum devised by Mutis and Isla. It established that students should visit the sick in the hospital and write a clinical history of each case; they should also perform autopsies. In addition the students were to assist in surgical operations whenever possible.

According to Isla:

> The study of theoretical medicine is to be contained in five school courses, as follows:
> The first year is to be devoted to theoretical anatomy at the School, and to hospital practice; the second year, to medical institutions; the third year, to

general and specific pathology; and the fourth and fifth years, to the Hippocratic doctrine.

Once these five years are completed, the students will be eligible to receive the degrees of their School. The practical experience in the Hospital will take three years; once completed, the physicians will receive their revalidation and their licence to practice.

The surgeons will undertake three years of theoretical and practical studies at the Hospital: The first year will be devoted to Anatomy; the second year, to surgical institutions; and the third year, to the practical study of operations.

Once these years are completed, they may be admitted to an examination and may obtain a license to practice.

Seven students registered for the first year, and the following textbooks were recommended for the first two years of study: Heister for anatomy; Boerhaave for physiology; and Haller for theory and introduction to medicine. During the third year they would study the treatise on *Morbis* by Boerhaave; in the fourth, the works of Hippocrates with comments by Parta, as well as the treatises on the air, water, and the atmosphere by Hippocrates; in the fifth, the *Medicaments* by Boerhaave, together with any new works by Murray and Cullen; the elementary principles of chemistry by Lavoiser and Chaptal, as well as any work new by Fourcroy. Botanical science was to be based on the writings of Ortega y Palau. Finally the students were required to read Switen van Hoffmann, Cullen, Morton, Gorter, Quarin, Haen, and, especially, Ramazini and Tizot, as well as the dictionary by James and the reports of the Faculty of Medicine in Paris.

Requests for admission to the school continued to increase each year.

In 1804 Mutis, Isla, and Caicedo introduced curricular reforms requiring, among other things, that every prospective candidate should have a knowledge of modern physics, mechanics, statics, and hydraulics. Chemistry, pharmacy, and botany would be studied during the apprenticeship period. Thursdays would be devoted to the practice of dissections at the hospital. Once the course on anatomy was concluded, surgery would follow, the teaching to be conducted on corpses. This would complete the first year. Physiology would be studied in the second year.

During the third there would be a course on pathology, and the students would visit the hospital. Then they would read *Sanitasis Tuenda* and *Methodo Modendi* by Boerhaave. Once pathology was completed, they would study diagnosis and prognosis, hygiene, and, finally, therapeutics. After passing the third-year examinations, the students would read the works of Hippocrates, starting with the *Principles*.

During the fifth year Boerhaave's *Viribus Medicamentorum* and *Materia Medica*, as well as chemistry and botany, would be studied. At the completion of the fifth year, students would receive the bachelor degree. They could then proceed to a hospital to practice for three years, taking clinical histories and studying Boerhaave's *De cognocendis et curandis morbis*, with commentary by van Hoffman. They would also study the *Principles of Surgery* by Boerhaave and the *Operations of Surgery* by Heister.

The first thesis to be printed was that of Joaquín Cagiao.

Isla died on 11 June 1807, and Tejada was appointed to replace him. In the same year, the government of Spain decided that the schools of medicine, surgery, and pharmacy were to be independent of each other.

The study plan of Mutis and Isla constituted a very important advancement in the study of medicine in Colombia: it was not simply a matter of reading; the courses were distributed among thoughtfully organized subjects. The requirements of hospital practice and dissections were established, as was the careful elaboration of clinical histories; in addition was the requirement that students study basic sciences such as chemistry, physics, and botany.

Tejada held the professorship until the War of Independence started. He graduated several disciples, but as he did not sympathize with the patriotic cause he suspended the courses and left for the Cauca.

In summarizing the study of medical teaching during colonial times in New Granada, we find several points of interest:

- Teaching was begun not long after the conquest had been concluded.
- The professorship was discontinued many times partly due to the lack of a physician to take it over and partly because of the scant interest of young men in medicine, as it was not considered a desirable career except for the less-favored classes. As a consequence, very few doctors were trained in Colombia.
- Teaching was centralized; there was no teaching of medicine outside the city of Santa Fé.
- At the end of the colonial era important modifications in teaching emerged, and requirements were established for certain scientific procedures that were different from the usual ones. This was the first and greatest reform, and perhaps the most important throughout the history of medicine in Colombia.

MEDICAL EDUCATION IN LATIN AMERICA: A BRIEF REVIEW

Gabriel Velazquez Palau

MEDICAL EDUCATION IN COLONIAL TIMES

In this brief essay on medical education in Latin America, I shall restrict myself to a few references to the colonial period and then talk about the changes that have occurred during the last twenty years. It is only natural that, because of my personal knowledge, I shall give more details about the changes that have taken place in Colombia.

The first universities in Latin America follow the Spanish pattern, with the influence of the University of Salamanca being particularly evident. Some were the result of "royal letters patent" (*cédulas reales*), which clearly showed the participation of the Catholic church since they were created by papal bulls and developed by religious communities. The first university was founded in 1538 in Santo Domingo by a decree of Pope Paul III; it was controlled by the Dominicans.

In May 1551 the University of San Marcos was established in Lima. It is interesting to note that between 1571 and 1583 the university had three rectors, all of whom were physicians who encouraged the teaching of medicine.

On 21 September 1551, by a royal letter patent of Charles V, Antonio de Mendoza, first viceroy of New Spain (Mexico) founded the Royal and Pontifical University of Mexico and entrusted the Franciscans with the teaching of medicine.

In Ecuador the Augustinians founded the University of San Fulgencio of Quito in 1586, authorized by a papal bull of Sixtus V. It did not begin to function until 1603, however, and medicine was not taught until 1693.

Although hospitals had been in operation since 1513, in Santa Maria del Darién, Cartagena, Santa Marta, and Santa Fé de Bogotá, it was not until 1636 that the lawyer and chief physician Rodrigo Enríquez de Andrade, authorized by the Jesuit rector, began to teach in the Dominicans' School of Santo Domingo in Santa Fé. Teaching had to be suspended for four years, however, for lack of students. In December 1653 Fray Cristóbal de Torres obtained permission to found the Superior College of Our Lady of the Rosary, availing himself of the royal letter patent that Philip IV had signed in 1651 authorizing the archbishop of Santa Fé to found a school to teach medicine in the kingdom of New Granada.

In the report rendered to the Spanish government in 1802, the illustrious physician José Celestino Mutis suggested a radical change in the medical curriculum by expanding it to eight years: five of theoretical studies in the medical school and three practical years in the hospital, with the student writing detailed essays on the subjects for each year. His plan called for prior preparation in mathematics and physics, and for the need to prepare native personnel who were familiar with the characteristic medical problems of the country.

It should be mentioned here that when the Harvard University was founded in 1636 fourteen universities were already in existence and operating in the Spanish possessions of Latin America.

In Central America the university of San Carlos de Guatemala, founded in 1676 by a royal letter patent of Charles II, opened its doors in January 1681, and the first class in medicine was inaugurated by Nicholas de Souza in October of the same year.

The Royal University of San Felipe was founded in San Ildefonso, Chile, in 1738 by a royal letter patent signed by Philip V. Medical studies were initiated in 1757. The university was closed in 1839. Andrés Bello prepared the bill for the law that in 1832 created what is today the University of Chile; Bello became its first rector. The university curriculum has included the teaching of medicine since its beginning.

The School of Santa Rosa was founded in Venezuela in 1661, but medical education did not begin until 1763 at the University of Caracas, when Lorenzo Campins y Ballester taught the first class.

In 1799 Charles IV authorized Viceroy Vertiz in Argentina to establish the first school of medicine in Buenos Aires, which was presided over by Miguel Gorman, an Irish physician and the first to teach medicine there.

It is interesting to point out that the *protomédicatus*, an institution that was established in Spanish America in the sixteenth century, had clearly defined duties that are still being analyzed in many countries. Their purposes were to maintain high levels of professional practice and specialization through the application of accrediting tests; to certify physicians, surgeons, pharmacists, and phlebotomists; and to examine the applicants for the licenciate and doctor's degree in medicine. The *protomédicatus* certified and authorized the sale of drugs; inspected pharmacies; controlled professional practice; and imposed fines for the illegal practice of medicine.

The first school of medicine in Brazil was founded in 1808; in 1910 only three were in existence; since 1950 their number has increased, perhaps too rapidly, to ninety.

THE ROLE OF SCIENTIFIC EXPEDITIONS

When reviewing the history of medical education in Latin America it is essential to mention, if only briefly, the role of the scientific expeditions that were organized by the Spanish Crown for the purpose of setting up an inventory of the natural resources of its colonies. In addition to obtaining very valuable information, these expeditions brought researchers of great prestige to America and encouraged interest in scientific research.

The *protomédicus* Francisco Hernández headed the first of these expeditions, which left for Mexico in the year 1570. In addition to his research on Mexican flora and fauna, which was published in seventeen volumes, this eminent physician and naturalist deserves to be mentionnd for his translation into Spanish of the thirty-seven volumes of the *Natural History of Cayus Plinius the Second*.

Peter Loefling took part in the expedition that Iturriaga and Alvarado made to Venezuela in the middle of the eighteenth century. Upon Loefling's death a few years later, his teacher, Carolus Linnaeus, the illustrious naturalist, published his diary and the *Flora Cumanensis*.

Charles III promoted several botanical expeditions, including those of Hipólito Ruiz and José Pavón who, between 1777 and 1788, explored Peru and Chile, where they collected and studied very valuable material. Ruiz, particularly, made numerous and important studies of how the American Indians utilized plants for medicinal purposes.

In 1783 another expedition was organized in New Granada. It was headed by the physician Mutis. Other prominent citizens of New Granada who joined this expedition included Francisco José de Caldas, Jorge Tadeo Lozano, Francisco Antonio Zea, and José Manuel Restrepo. This voyage was probably one of the most valuable and productive: over 6,000 specimens of plants were collected; the traditional use of *quina* (quinine or Cinchona bark) by the Indians in New Granada was described; and many highly accurate drawings of great scientific and artistic value were made.

The third expedition was largely due to the private initiative of Martín Sessé, a physician from Aragón, who, as a great admirer of Francisco Hernández and his work, decided to continue it. His advisor was the Mexican physician, José María Mocino, and together they collected a wealth of material and published such works as *Flora Mexicana* and *Plantae Novae Hispaniae*.

In 1789 the so-called Malaspina expedition left to explore the vast regions of Argentina, Uruguay, Chile, Panama, and Mexico, and went on thereafter to Guam, Australia, and the Philippines.

Another major expedition was the so-called vaccination expedition of Balmis to Venezuela, Colombia, Ecuador, Peru, Bolivia, Mexico, and Central America. This took place at the beginning of the nineteenth century and is very well described in this volume by Ricardo Archila.

DEVELOPMENT OF MEDICAL EDUCATION

In Colombia, and in Latin America in general, four very characteristic periods can be identified in the development of medical education.

- During colonial times teaching was largely carried out through the private initiative of Spanish physicians authorized by royal letters patent or papal bulls. Assisted by religious communities they organized rather scattered classes that were either interrupted or suspended quite frequently.

- At the end of the colonial period medical schools were organized and founded in state-supported and private universities and colleges. Training at these institutions was interrupted by the wars of independence and the civil wars that followed.

- At the end of the nineteenth century and at the beginning of the present one, the universities and medical schools were organized in a more stable manner, following in general the old European pattern, particularly that of the French.

- Since 1950 very accelerated reforms in the educational systems have been started in various countries of Latin America. These reforms have produced enormous changes in virtually all countries during the last twenty years.

THE LAST TWENTY YEARS

During the first half of the present century the curriculum in Latin American medical schools was almost an exact copy of the French curriculum; the literature and most of the textbooks were written in French; postgraduate training was taken in France; the majority of the professors had spent some time in that country; and several French missions visited Colombia and other Latin American countries.

The Second World War and the invasion of France by the Germans interrupted that exchange, with the result that communication with North America became increasingly more intensive. A great number of scholarships were given to Latin American physicians to study in the United States; initially, young doctors, and later, professors, went there frequently; and, as English-language literature became more accessible, there was more communication with other countries such as Canada and Great Britain. During the last ten years a noticeable exchange of ideas and programs among Latin American medical educators themselves has contributed to the creation of what may be called the Latin American school or approach.

A common characteristic of this movement is a concern for aspects of preventive medicine, which in several countries has led to the development of extramural programs of family medicine, whereby medical, nursing, and dental students take part in experimental programs to furnish health services to communities, and health aides and promoters are trained to assume preventive and healing tasks.

At the beginning of 1950, in Colombia and other countries of Latin America, the following features prevailed in university structure and in medical education, almost all of them inherited from Europe, especially France:

- The structure and integration of the universities were very weak. Traditionally the university was the result of groupings of schools or colleges, among which there was very little communication. Their administration was unstable, being composed of part-time deans or directors who had inadequate preparation for their positions.
- The faculty was made up primarily of practicing clinicians who devoted a few hours a week to teaching. Teaching of the basic medical sciences was especially poor. Great emphasis was placed on didactic lectures, and the laboratories usually lacked sufficient equipment for practical instruction.
- The curriculum consisted of thirty-five to forty completely uncoordinated courses, which resulted in unnecessary duplications, and, even worse, the omission of important subjects. Clinical instruction was poor, with an excessive number of theoretical classes being given at a patient's bedside. All teaching was carried out within the medical school, and the

students were unaware of the health problems of the surrounding community. Internships, residencies, and graduate training did not exist. Very little research was carried on. Student enrollments were frequently excessive, and the admissions systems, when they existed, were inadequate and applied without any scientific criteria.

Over the past twenty years these deficiencies have been corrected in several Latin American medical schools. In many countries, particularly Brazil, Chile, Peru, Venezuela, and Colombia, interesting reforms and innovations in the structure and orientation of medical education are being tried out successfully. Because I am more familiar with them, I will summarize the major changes that have taken place in the medical school of Del Valle University in Cali.

The report of the medical mission headed by Dr. G.H. Humphreys, which was sent by the United States Unitarian Service Committee to Colombia in 1948, had great influence on the creation of this school. Also evident was the impact on Colombian medical schools of the visit and the recommendations of the North America medical mission made up of Drs. Max E. Lapham, Robert Berson, and Charles Goss, who visited Colombia in 1953.

Organization and Scientific Development: 1951-55

With the cooperation of the W.K. Kellogg and Rockefeller foundations, a fellowship program was initiated for the continuing education of professors of medicine; between 1951 and 1955 over thirty professors traveled abroad. Upon their return a full-time faculty system was set up, thus breaking away from the old part-time tradition; the basic and clinical sciences were strengthened; the previous system of uncoordinated classes was replaced by teaching departments that grouped related subjects together; more importance was placed on practical teaching in the laboratories; and clinical clerkships at the patient's bedside were introduced. The humanities were integrated into the medical curriculum; the number of students per class was limited to sixty; and a strict admissions system was established.

Teaching Preventive Medicine and Public Health: 1955-60

Great attention continued to be given to the development of the basic and clinical sciences through constant endeavors to update the faculty's training. As of 1971, over 160 professors had received fellowships to prepare as teachers and researchers.

During this particular period attention was given to the development of a solid program in preventive and family medicine, through the creation of a strong Department of Preventive Medicine and Public Health. Pilot programs for research and teaching were established in the low-income districts of Cali and in the rural zone of Candelaria. The teaching of these disciplines was extended throughout the medical school years. Students worked in extramural programs, thereby developing the concepts and principles of integrated medical care and family preventive medicine in a practical manner. During this period, also, the administration was improved and reinforced; the dean, the associate deans, and all department heads became full-time faculty members.

Community Research: 1960-66

In the early 1960s some professors began to become aware of the need to organize programs that would allow them to teach systems directed not only toward the solution of problems of the sick individual, but toward the promotion of the health of the family and the community. More attention was given to the study of socioeconomic and cultural factors that would lead to a better understanding of the needs of both urban and rural population groups. Basic, clinical, and applied research projects were developed intensively. Numerous field studies were introduced to learn more about the health problems of Colombia, as well as about the available resources, methods, and techniques with which to solve them.

Professors and students took an active part in the planning and development of the Study of Human Resources for Health and Medical Education, which was initiated in 1964 under the joint direction of the Colombian Association of Medical Schools and the Ministry of Health. In the course of the study, research was conducted on numerous factors related to health; analyses were made of possible solutions to such problems as the high population growth rate, unemployment, lack of education, migration, overcrowded housing, lack of drinking water, and waste disposal; and studies were made of the impact of these problems on the health of the population.

The need for a multidisciplinary team approach became increasingly more apparent. The first teams to adopt this approach consisted of professors and students of nursing, dentistry, sanitary engineering, architecture, and economics, in addition to professors and students of medicine.

Creation of the Health Division: 1966-71

Parallel to the foregoing developments in the medical school, other units of Del Valle University underwent similar changes. The economics department became interested in the study of landholding, land use, and production and agricultural marketing problems; the architecture division looked into housing and the construction of low-cost dwellings; the engineering school made studies of adequate systems of drinking water and waste disposal, and the possibility of accelerating the industrial development process.

Out of all these activities the conviction was born that one of the main missions of a university is to contribute to the promotion and acceleration of the development and welfare of the people in its community. To achieve this goal it should prepare the leaders of tomorrow; take part in research on community problems and try to find solutions to them; and offer advice and services to agencies in the region. To facilitate achievement of these objectives Del Valle University was reorganized: its schools, divisions, and related academic units were regrouped, and the concept of the Division of Health Sciences was born.

The division incorporated the medical school's undergraduate and graduate programs; the nursing school's programs for master's and licenciate degrees, and for registered nurses, nurses' aides, and health promoters; the clinical technology laboratory; the physiotherapy and rehabilitation school; and the stomatology department. For its academic program the division receives the cooperation of the schools of engineering, economics, and education, and takes an active part in three multidisciplinary university centers: the Center for Population Research, the Multidisciplinary Research Center on Social Systems, and the Resource Center for Education and Teaching.

In conclusion it should be mentioned for the record that the National Associations of Medical Schools and the Panamerican Federation of Associations of Medical Schools both had a great influence on the development of medical education in Latin America during the 1960s.

TWO FOOTNOTES TO COLONIAL MEDICAL HISTORY: The *Regimento* of Guilherme Escoph de Esens, and the *Erario Mineral* of Luís Gomes Ferreira, 1733 and 1735

Charles R. Boxer

THE *REGIMENTO* OF GUILHERME ESCOPH DE ESENS—1639

I cannot find any reference to this author or to his *Regimento* in any of the standard bibliographies of medical history.[1] The only copy I have been able to find is in the Public Library at Ponta Delgada, São Miguel, Azores, although I suspect there must be copies in other Portuguese libraries. This treatise is obviously extremely rare and I am grateful to the director of the library at Ponta Delgada and to my friend, Senhor Anibal Cymbron Barbosa Bettencourt, for their kindness in supplying me with a copy.

Judging from the wording of the title page, the author was probably a German from Essen. Except for that and the dedication to Luís Cesar I have no information about him. In translation, the title page reads:

> Instruction concerning the application of the remedies that are carried in the medicine chests (*boticas*) that are embarked in any galleon or other ship on His Majesty's service. Something very necessary in order to prevent the sick from dying for want of someone who knows how to apply them. Dedicated to Luís Cesar, Superintendent of the Magazines and Fleets of the Kingdom of

Portugal. By Guilherme Escoph de Esens, qualified physician, surgeon, and apothecary, and surgeon of His Majesty; Chief Surgeon of the Galleys of the Kingdom of Portugal. *With licence.* In Lisbon, by Jorge Rodrigues. Anno 1639.

In the dedication to Cesar the author apologizes for having had to compile the work in such a hurry and for his grammatical errors as a foreigner. The civil ecclesiastical licenses to print the volume are dated between 13 April and 4 May 1639, an unusually speedy passage for a book at that period, and they include two that read as follows:

> The King Our Lord orders that the Chief Physician (*Fisico Mòr*) should examine this instruction concerning the medicine chests that are embarked for regions overseas, and state his opinion thereof, which he will do with all dispatch. Lisbon, 16 April 1639. *Sebastião de Carvalho. Balthasar Fialho.*

and

> I examined this treatise of remedies, both internal and external, and others that are quintessential, the which are usefully and studiously compiled by Guilherme Escoph de Esens and are very necessary for those who sail in His Majesty's ships, since very often they do not carry qualified physicians and surgeons; and this is a brief compilation instructing how to apply the remedies that they carry; and thus I am of the opinion that it can be printed. Lisbon, 16 April 1639. *The Chief Surgeon, Simão Roubão da Costa.*

The *Regimento* was thus intended for general use in all the ships of the Crown of Portugal in the Atlantic and in the Asian seas. Possibly the reason for the haste with which it was compiled was that copies were intended for use in the Portuguese Squadron of the combined armada of Don Antonio de Oquendo, which was being prepared that summer and which was destroyed by the Dutch Admiral M.H. Tromp in the battle of the Downs on 21 October 1639.[2]

The contents are divided into two parts: The first begins by listing the "external remedies," which are subdivided into various categories such as *unguentos* (ointments); emprastos (plasters); *oleos* and *azeites* (oils); *cataplasmas* (poultices); *collirios* (eye salves); *banhos* (lotions and distilled waters); and *pós* (powders); some of these are further subdivided. Then follows a list of the "internal remedies" grouped under the subheadings of *xaropes* (syrups); *conservas* (conserves or comfits); *electuarios* (electuaries); *pirolas* (pills); *cordeais* (cordials); *opiatis* (opiates); *simples internos* (internal simples); and *agoas internas* (internal waters). This list of contents is followed by a brief description of the therapeutic qualities of each of the seventy-six remedies, usually accompanied by a brief statement of how they should be applied or used, beginning with *Unguento Rozado* and ending with *Theriaga Magna de Andromachi.*

The second part begins with a heading that reads:

Instruction concerning the extraordinary remedies that are additionally embarked in these medicine chests; made and prepared by my own hand, and which can be used with confidence because I have had much experience in using them in various lands, and in diseases that many physicians and surgeons had despaired of curing; with which I always achieved good and happy results. There is a most certain thing, and the shortest cure that can be effected in any new or old wound, in bullet wounds, gunpowder burns, [boiling] oil, or in any other mishap.

Then follows a numbered list of seventeen additional remedies, with the ills they are supposed to cure; these are likewise subdivided into ten "external remedies" and seven "internal remedies." The remainder of the second part consists of a description of how each of these remedies should be applied, beginning with an *Emprasto com o qual sara todas as chagas ou feridas* (Plaster that heals all sores or wounds) and ending with a *Remedio contra o mal dos rins* (Remedy against disease of the kidneys). Some of these additional remedies are concerned with the cure of wounds, fistulas, and suppurating sores; others are offered as treatment for fevers, agues, jaundice, constipation, dysentery, and many other ills to which the flesh is heir by land and sea. I give two examples:

No. 4. Lotion Against the Worms of Brazil[3]

Anyone who suffers from this disease can apply this lotion, which is done as follows: rosewater, *tanchage* water, one white of an egg, and *aluayade* powder. Mix ingredients very well, and when they begin to swell after having been well stirred, take a piece of cloth moistened in this lotion and apply it three or four times a day to the infected part, and likewise after every time that the patient goes to stool, and he will be cured in a short time.

No. 17. Remedy for the Disease of the Kidneys

When a person cannot urinate, owing to a stoppage in the urinal veins, due to vescosities, or gravel, or any other mishap which might befall the kidneys, or from smallpox, take three or four drops of this oil mixed with two or three spoonfuls of wine, and drink this dosage every morning for six or seven days in succession. The patient will soon find himself to be very much better, God willing.

God willing (*Deos querendo*) does indeed seem the *mot juste* here and in others of these remedies.

It is interesting to compare the seventy-six remedies listed in this *Regimento* of 1639 with the contents of an English naval surgeon's medical chest in the same year, as illustrated in John Woodall's *The Surgeon's Mate*.[4] Some earlier and later Portuguese lists of the contents of medicine chests for shipboard use, compiled between 1519 and 1744, can be found in the following works:

1519. Américo Pires de Lima, "A botica de bordo de Fernão de Magalhães," *Anais da Faculdade de Farmácia do Porto* IV (1957).

1617. "Roi da Botica que foi para Moçambique na Urca *Cavallo Marinho,"* published with a valuable commentary by Américo Pires de Lima in "Como se tratavam os Portugueses em Moçambique, no primeiro quartel do século XII," *Anais da Faculdade de Farmácia do Porto* II (1941).

1631. António de Ataide, "Botica para a gente de mar de hũa Nao da Índia, a qual quando ha contratador dos mantimentos vaj incluido no contrato." António de Ataide papers, Houghton Library, Harvard University. Published in C.R. Boxer, "The *Carreira da India:* Ships, Men, Cargoes, Voyages," reprinted from *O Centro de Estudos Históricas Ultramarinos e as Commemorações Henriquinas* (Lisbon) no. 1744 (1961).

1744. Pedro de Almeida (Conde de Castello-Novo and Viceroy of India), "Relaçáo dos medicamentos com que se proveo a botica da fragata *Nossa Senhora a Madre de Deos* que na prezente monção de 1744 voy para o Estado de India." Pedro de Almeida Papers. In C.R. Boxer, "Moçambique Island and the *Carreira da India,* reprinted from *Studia Revista Semestral* (Lisbon) no. 8 (1961).

A further comparison can be made with the contents of Dutch naval medicine and surgeons' chests in the seventeenth century, in the light of those reproduced and analyzed in the works of A. Leuftink.[5] Not being a medical historian I will not presume to make an analytical comparison, but there are two general observations a layman may be permitted to make.

Pires de Lima has remarked that there was relatively little difference between the *boticas* carried by the ships of Magalhães's fleet in 1519 and those sent to Moçambique almost exactly a century later. Similarly, Leuftink has observed that the contents of the Dutch surgeon's chest in 1692 varied little from that recommended at the beginning of that century. The inherently conservative nature of both the seaman's calling and the medical profession during that period probably contributed to this state of affairs, although of course no really major advances could have been expected before the time of the great scientific discoveries of the nineteenth century.

One other observation is suggested by the *Regimento:* Sir Richard Hawkins, in his *Observations* of 1622, criticized the Spaniards and, by implication, the Portuguese—since the two Iberian crowns were united between 1580 and 1640—for being "nothing so curious in accommodating themselves with good and careful surgeons, nor to fit them with that which belongeth to their profession, as other nations are, though they have greater need than I do know."⁶ The criticism was not entirely fair. The *Instrucción de Generales y Almirantes de Flotas de la Carreira de Indias*, promulgated at El Escorial on 7 June 1597, left the nursing of the sick and wounded to the "clergy and religious (*clerigos y religiosos*) who will sail in all the fleets." But further on the *Instrucción* became rather more specific and implied that a qualified physician or medical doctor was also taken along:

> If there are sick in the ships of the fleet, great attention must be paid to them, and they must be given all the medicines the doctor orders, and the food and diet from the things which are provided for this purpose and which are carried on board the said ships; and the General and the Comptroller will take great care that these are not consumed in other ways, lest they be found wanting in an emergency. And from the day the sick man is placed on a diet, the Comptroller and the ration clerk will take care to enter him in their books, so that the master does not give him another ration, nor will he be credited with the same even if he claims he issued it.

The *Ordenanzas para el Buen Gobierno de la Armada Real del Mar Oceano*, promulgated on 24 January 1633, replaced the *Instrucción* of 1597 and made much more detailed arrangements for the care of the sick and wounded; presumably it was used in the armada of the Crown of Portugal also.⁷ Among other things, provision was made for the use of hospital ships, although this was not exactly an innovation since two had sailed in the armada of 1588. As J.J. Keevil admits, this was certainly more advanced than the contemporary English naval organization, and it is odd that Hawkins should have ignored it.⁸ Admittedly, theory ran ahead of practice in both the *Instrucción* of 1597 and the *Ordenanzas* of 1633, since complaints of the lack or inefficiency of shipboard medical and surgical care abounded during this period. The *clerigos y religiosos* principally concerned with nursing the sick and wounded in the Spanish armadas, *flotas*, and shore hospitals, where these existed, were the friars or regular clergy of the Order of San Juan de Dios. Their contribution can be gauged from the work of Salvador Clavijo y Clavijo.⁹ The Portuguese seem rather to have relied on Franciscan shipboard chaplains who doubled in nursing the sick, as did the Jesuits and other religious in the Portuguese East-Indiamen. But the friars of São João de Deos, as the Portuguese branch of the order was called, began to play a more prominent and regular role from the 1690s onward.¹⁰

The *boticas* laid down in the *Regimento* of 1639 and elsewhere were also used ashore. Here again there was much contemporary criticism of the total lack or inadequacy of hospitalization for the sick and wounded from fleets and ships. In the *Diálogo entre un Vizcaíno y un Montanés* a horrifying picture is drawn of the enormous death rate among military and naval personnel in Spanish seaports for lack of hospitals in which to treat them in the period 1590 to 1630.¹¹ The anonymous writer is particularly scandalized by the contrast between the generously endowed hospitals for the relief of the vagabond poor and the total absence of them for far more deserving service personnel:

> ... and it is a lamentable thing that in Madrid, Seville, and other great places of Spain, there are holy hospitals, so large and with such fine endowments, where so many vagabonds who are a scandal to God and to the common weal are treated and cured; while for those who serve His Majesty and sustain his monarchy and the Catholic Church, there is not a hospital that will treat them, nor a pious individual who will leave a remembrance for such a just and holy purpose; whereas there are so many persons who will bequeath their estates to hospitals that give shelter and treatment to people of the aforesaid kind. His Majesty should maintain one [naval] hospital in Pasaje, another in Santander, another in Ferrol or in Coruña, another in Lisbon, and another in Cadiz, which are the ports where the fleets are fitted out . . . . ¹²

This is somewhat exaggerated as there was at least one naval hospital, the Hospital de las Galeras de la Iglesia de San Juan de Letrán in Puerto de Santa María, which functioned from 1587 onward. Nevertheless it is indisputable that in all western countries with overseas possessions in the seventeenth century there was seldom adequate hospital treatment available for service personnel. One of the few exceptions, for part of the time at any rate, was the Royal Hospital in Goa, so enthusiastically described in the early seventeenth century by the French sailor, François Pyrard de Laval.¹³ There does not seem to have been any hospital quite so spacious and well furnished in contemporary colonial America, although this is a point on which I would not like to be dogmatic.¹⁴

Reverting to Portuguese, as distinct from Spanish, maritime medical practice, each Indiaman was supposed to carry a qualified physician and a surgeon, together with well-stocked medicine chests provided by the crown. As we have seen from the wording of the 1639 *Regimento*, however, in actual fact there was often a dearth or a total absence of qualified medical personnel.¹⁵ For example, in the India fleet of 1633, which carried 3,000 men in four ships, there was only an ignorant barber-surgeon in each ship. Toward the end of the seventeenth century repeated complaints were received in Lisbon from Goa about the lack of qualified doctors in the Indiamen, and the disinclination of the nursing orderlies to care for the sick properly for fear of catching infection. The Viceroy of India suggested in 1698 that friars of the nursing order of São João de Deos should be asked to act as ships' doctors. He proposed that two friars should sail in each East-Indiaman, and that they should have under their supervision four male nurses to take care of the sick. This suggestion was adopted for a time and the friars seem to have given great satisfaction, as they were already doing in their small but well-run hospital in Moçambique.[16]

It is clear that the crown in the sixteenth, seventeenth, and eighteenth centuries was generous with the provision of well-stocked medicine chests to each East-Indiaman, but all too often the contents were embezzled by unauthorized persons for their own use or were sold for profit on the ship's black market instead of being freely distributed to the sick. These continuing abuses help to explain why there was no decline in the high mortality rate that prevailed in the outward-bound Portuguese Indiamen for most of the seventeenth and eighteenth centuries. It can also be seen that many of the medicinal drugs listed in the 1639 and other *Regimentos* had little or no therapeutic value.

But the main reason for the continuing high mortality rate was the fact that so many of the convict-soldiers who embarked at Lisbon were already infected with typhus and other diseases, which spread rapidly in the overcrowded conditions aboard ship.[17] The mortality in the Brazil fleets was much lower because the voyage was so much shorter, and because fewer *degredados* (jailbirds) were aboard.[18] The *Regimento* of 1639 furnishes additional proof that if the Portuguese crown failed to cope with the menace presented by disease on voyages in tropical waters it did try to take such remedial measures as the limited scientific knowledge of the age allowed.

THE *ERARIO MINERAL* OF LUÍS GOMES FERREIRA, 1735 and 1755

This outstanding work on Luso-Brazilian medicine and surgery in the eighteenth century is known from two editions published in Lisbon in 1735 and 1755, respectively, both of which are very rare, especially the latter, of which I have been able to locate only one apparently complete copy; it was bought from a Lisbon bookseller by the Lilly Library of Indiana University in 1969. This two-volume edition has been described by me in some detail elsewhere.[19]* A tentative comparison was made with the 1735 edition, but, as I could not find a copy of it anywhere in the United States or the United Kingdom at the time, I was unable to determine precisely in what way the contents of the two editions differed. The Lilly Library having recently

---

* Shortly after publication of that article Francisco Guerra advised me that a copy of volume 2 of the 1755 edition is held by the Faculty of Medicine in Lisbon, and is listed in the catalogue of its library compiled by M. Athias: *Catálogo das Obras da Colecção Portuguesa Anteriories à Fundação das Régias Escolas de Cirurgia em 1825* (Lisbon: n.p., 1942): 138. I am very grateful to this illustrious medical historian for this information.

acquired a copy of the first edition, I have now been able to make a page-by-page comparison, with the result I shall describe.

Both the author and the publisher claimed that the 1755 edition was a greatly expanded version of the first. The title pages of the two 1755 volumes state: "Now reprinted and enlarged with a great number of exquisite and wonderful prescriptions." The author's *Proemio* explains that it was being published in a two-volume format owing to its greatly expanded contents.

In 1969 I ventured the tentative suggestion that the additional matter was mainly if not entirely confined to *Tratado III, Da Miscellania*, an assortment of cures, remedies, and prescriptions for a great variety of diseases, most of which resembled old wives' and quack doctors' nostrums. This suggestion turned out to be correct. Apart from some minor rearrangements of wording in the preliminary matter and lists of contents, the additional textual matter is placed in the *Tratado III, Da Miscellania*. In the 1735 edition this section ends with a piece entitled "Remedios, para que os bebedos aborreção o vinho" (Remedies to make drunkards dislike wine). In the 1755 edition this piece is followed by a "Collirio para queixas dos ólhos" (Eye salve for complaints of the eyes), and by another seventy-five recipes, cures, and prescriptions of the most varied and often fantastic description. A subhead following this section is entitled "Varios remedios avulsos, que obrão maravilhosamente com a sua virtude" (Various different remedies which work wonders with their virtue). This is followed by another eighteen assorted recipes, cures, and prescriptions. The total additional matter therefore consists of some ninety-three remedies on thirty-one pages.

These additions vary in length from a couple of pages to a couple of lines, but most of them are very short. The longest is on the preparation and application of quinine (*Preparação da quina quina*), and many others are concerned with cures for toothache. Their therapeutic value or lack of it can be judged by the following two extracts, which are by no means the most fantastic:

> The bone of a frog (of that kind which has a black spot) when touched against the aching tooth causes the pain to go at once.
> The root of the mallow, placed against the aching tooth when the pain is acute, will cause it to go at once.

Other cures, remedies, and prescriptions in this additional section deal with wounds, venereal diseases, worms, retention of urine, intermittent fevers, epilepsy, and so on. Much is made of the marvelous therapeutic properties of a complicated nostrum, *Espirito Angelico*, which is recommended as a virtual cure-all for such varied complaints as headache, sore eyes, earache, toothache, old and new wounds, and cuts and contusions, to name only a few of the ills listed—"In all these cases it has been tried with success many times."

It is not fair to judge Luís Gomes Ferreira's *Erario Mineral* by his advocacy of such primitive folk medicine, but, as I noted in my article,[20] it is rather surprising that he continued to advocate such cures after his return to the flourishing city of Oporto from the backlands of Minas Gerais.

Many of these additional remedies are indexed at the end of Volume 2 of the 1755 edition, otherwise it is basically the same as that in the 1735 edition, except of course for the changes in page references.

In conclusion I may add that the thirteen unnumbered preliminary pages of laudatory poems and sonnets addressed to Luís Gomes Ferreira by some of his friends in the 1735 edition are omitted in that of 1755. In any event they are not present in the Lilly Library copy, which appears to be complete, although it lacks the mandatory civil and ecclesiastical licenses. Clarifications must await the location of another copy of the first volume, which has so far eluded bibliographers.

NOTES

1. The same is true of relevant articles on medical history by Portuguese specialists in this field, such as Augusto da Silva Carvalho, Américo Pires de Lima, and Luís de Pina, although there is one article by de Pina that I have not seen: "La Médicine Maritime Portugaise dans les 16 et 17 siècles," in *Atti del XVIII Congreso Nazionale di Storia della Medicina* (Rome: n.p., 1962).
2. C.R. Boxer, ed. and transl., *The Journal of Maarten Harpertszoon Tromp Anno 1639* (Cambridge: Cambridge University Press, 1930).
3. For the various diseases included in this portmanteau term, see Francisco Guerra, "Aleixo de Abreu, 1568-1630. Author of the Earliest Book on Tropical Medicine, Describing Amoebiasis, Malaria, Typhoid Fever, Yellow Fever, Dracontiasis, Trichuriasis, and Tungiasis in 1623," *Journal of Tropical Medicine and Hygiene* 71 (March 1968): 55-69.
4. John Woodall, *The Surgeon's Mate* (London: n.p., 1639). See the plan showing the contents of Woodall's sea surgeon's chest reproduced between pages 200 and 201 in J.J. Keevil, *Medicine and the Navy*, 1200-1900, vol. I, 1200-1649, and his comments on pp. 198-99 and 218 (Edinburgh and London: E. & S. Livingstone, Ltd., 1957).
5. A. Leuftink, *De Geneeskunde bij's Lands oorlogsvloot in de 17e eeuw* (Assen: Van Gorcum, 1953); and idem, *De Chirurgijns zee-compas: de medische verzorging aan boord van Nederlandsche zeeschepen gedurende de Gouden Eeuw* (Baarn: n.p., 1963).
6. Sir Richard Hawkins, *Obervations* (London: I. Iaggard, 1622): 159.
7. It is included in J.J. Andrade e Silva, *Collecção Chronológica de legislação antiga Portugueza, 1627-1633*. (Lisbon: F.X. de Sousa, 1855): 259-306. The relevant paragraphs are reproduced in Salvador Clavijo y Clavijo, *La Trayectoria Hospitalaria de la Armada Española* (Madrid: Instituto Histórico de la Marina, 1944): 23-25.
8. Keevil, *Medicine and the Navy* (See note 4).
9. Salvador Clavijo y Clavijo, *La Ordeu Hospitalaria de San Juan de Dios en la Mariña de*

guerra de España, Presencia y nexo, 1550-1950, especially "La Hospitalidad de San Juan de Dios navegando por las aguas de los dominios Hispanomericanos, siglo XVII" (Madrid: Tipografia Artistica, 1950): 143-78.

10. António Alberto de Andrade, *Os Hospitaleiros de São João de Deos no ultramar. Subsidios para a sua história* (Lisbon: F.X. de Sousa, 1957). It was said of these friars in 1680-81, ". . . so elles sambem ter cuidado dos enfermos e tratar da saude delles."

11. Written circa 1635-40, the *Diálogo* was first published by Cesareo Fernández Duro, *Disquisiciones Nauticas*, vol. VI (Madrid: n.p. 1881). Extracts appear in Clavijo y Clavijo, *La Trayectoria Hospitalaria* (See note 7).

12. Ibid.: 21-23.

13. First published in 1619, the best edition is that translated and edited by A. Gray and H.C. Bell, *Voyage of François Pyrard of Laval to the East Indies, the Maldives, the Moluccas and Brazil*, 3 vols. (London: Hakluyt Society, 1887-90).

14. Woodrow Borah, *Social Welfare and Social Obligation in New Spain: A Tentative Assessment* (Los Angeles: Center for Latin American Studies, University of California, reprint no. 282, n.d.).

15. Typical of these longstanding complaints is that of the anonymous writer of a newsletter from Goa in 1691: "And one of the reasons there is such heavy mortality, besides the fact that the ships leave very late, and thus their voyages last for seven months, is that no physicians sail in these ships. And it seems a kind of cruelty for our Lord the King to send a thousand Portuguese to this State, with the principal aim that they should arrive here alive and live for many years, yet no physicians are sent. . . ." (Novas da India, Janeiro 1691), in Panduronga Pissurlencar, *Assento do Conselho do Estado da India*, vol. V (Bastorá: Arquivo Histórico da Índia, 1957): 578.

16. The viceroy complained in a dispatch to the crown (Goa, 18 December 1698) that "the nursing orderlies, owing to their dread of becoming infected by the contagious diseases, abandon the sick, as I have reported," in "Documentos da Índia," Box 37, Arquivo Histórico Ultramarino, Lisbon. See also, A.A. de Andrade, "Fundação do Hospital Militar de São João de Deos em Moçambique," in *Studia Revista Semestral* (Lisbon) I (1961): 95-132, especially pp. 101-13 and the sources quoted therein.

17. As Padre Feruão de Queiroz, S.J., graphically explained in 1687: "Nor can many deaths be avoided in such a wide range of climates; for even though the sea is healthier than the land, there are many causes of infection: as can be seen in the stale, recooked, and rotten provisions; the drinking water in pipes whereof the wood has been ill cured, and still more so after passing the latitude of Guinea; in the infected convicts sent from the Limoeiro and Cabria prisons; in the crowd of people on board and the shortage of living space, so that if many fall sick the resultant and unavoidable lack of hygiene makes things still worse; in the distribution of rations that are unsuitable for the various climates; and other lesser evils; these are sufficient reasons for the loss of health and lives. And if the voyages are long and without refreshments, the ravages of scurvy are unavoidable " *Conquista Temporal e Espiritual de Ceylão*, livro VI, cap. 14 (Colombo: Ceylon Government Press, 1916): 908.

18. For the treatment in Bahia of the sick from outward- and homeward-bound Portuguese East-Indiamen, see A.J.R. Russell-Wood, *Fidalgos and Philanthropists: The Santa Casa da Misericórdia of Bahia, 1550-1755* (London: MacMillan and Co., 1968): 159, 263-93, passim.

19. C.R. Boxer, "A Rare Luso-Brazilian Medical Treatise and Its Author: Luís Gomes Ferreira and His *Erario Mineral* of 1735 and 1755," *Indiana University Bookman*, no. 10 (November 1969): 49-70. For a bibliographic description of the 1735 edition, see Rubens Borba de Moraes, *Bibliographica Brasiliana*, 2 vols. (Rio de Janeiro and Amsterdam: Colibris Editora, 1958): vol. 1, 262.

20. Boxer, ibid.

THE BALMIS EXPEDITION IN VENEZUELA. PART II: FOUNDING OF THE CENTRAL VACCINATION BOARD, 1804

Ricardo Archila

JUSTIFICATION

Among the many Spanish scientific expeditions that visited and explored the territories of the New World, those that stand out went beyond the continent, and, from the universal point of view, acquired the characteristics of a circumvolution. A forerunner of this type was the voyage of Alejandro Malaspina (1789-94), which unfortunately was frustrated because it went no further than the Philippines and some of the South Sea Islands.[1]

Circumscribed by this historical approach, there is no doubt that the first Spanish circumvoluted scientific expedition was the Royal Maritime Expedition, often called the "Balmis expedition" or the "vaccination expedition." It is significant that both Malaspina's and Balmis's voyages took place under the rule of Charles IV, during the period of Bourbon Spain.

In spite of the importance of the Balmis voyage—a chapter in the history of medicine and of science—more than a century was to pass until its true meaning became apparent and its purpose fulfilled.

This historical facts have been brought out thanks to a comprehensive bibliography that has tried to unravel and elucidate the objective, the itinerary, and the results obtained by the expedition.[2]

If objective justice were parallel to the historiographical contribution itself, the vaccination expedition would now be called "a closed case," in the language of the jurists. It continues to be "an open case," however, a topic of study and research for historians, because, first, the regions covered by the expedition are vast, and, second, although the relevant bibliography is extensive and valuable it does not contain the details of each place visited. In brief, no complete narrative or analytical history as yet exists on the subject. In those that have been written there is still relatively much to be investigated further. To date, for example, there is no knowledge of the whereabouts of the logbook the director of the expedition was compelled to keep, nor are its contents known.

Moreover, although the archives of the Indies have been explored exhaustively in this respect,[3] we assume that other historical sources or documentary repositories still exist in those countries that once comprised Spain's overseas empire, which could supply unpublished regional information. An example of this is the volume, *Expedición de la Vacuna*,[4] which is in the archives of the illustrious Municipal Council of the Federal District of Venezuela.

Thus it seems logical and timely to take advantage of this occasion to discuss Venezuela's contribution after the introduction of the smallpox vaccine in Venezuela by the Balmis expedition, as well as the tasks performed by the Central Vaccination Board.

FIRST STAGE: 1804–06

Creation of the Central Vaccination Board

The expedition stayed in Venezuela from 20 March to 8 May 1804. During that short interval, not only was mass vaccination introduced successfully in the cities of Caracas and Valencia and in the ports of La Guaira, Puerto Cabello, and Maracaibo, but Balmis had the satisfaction of establishing the Central Vaccination Board in Caracas. Two decisions of great importance were taken: the foundation of the board, and the ultimate subdivision of the expedition. The latter was a very necessary initiative, because only by branching out into two parts could it achieve its ambitious program.

Apparently Balmis had the Spanish government's approval of the project, based on the negative experiences he had observed in other parts of the old continent, where private enterprises ended in failure due to the lack of official backing. Naturally, he had received precise orders, among them the obligation to train physicians in the vaccination method along the route to be covered; to this end he had to supply them with copies of the Moreau de la Sarthe Treaty, which Balmis himself had translated in Paris in 1803. On the other hand, he was urged to obtain the cooperation of high ecclesiastical authorities everywhere—a reflection of the very powerful influence the church enjoyed at the time.

On his first stop, Santa Cruz de Tenerife, Balmis founded a "vaccination house"; in San Juan de Puerto Rico, he was unable to make any special arrangements. It was in Caracas, the third stop, that the crystalization of his idea occurred with the founding of a technical-administrative body for the purpose of complying with the basic objective, "to preserve, perpetuate and make appropriate use of the precious fluid," after the mission's departure. It should be pointed out in this respect that the stipulation and plans, as outlined previously in Spain,[5] were not always precisely followed; sometimes they were modified, particularly by the Council of the Indies.

That is what occurred in Venezuela with regard to the vaccination houses. When the Spanish monarch learned about the arrival of his envoys in the Indies he became so elated about the news of their successes that on 20 May 1804 he issued a royal order for the operation of vaccination wards in the hospitals of the capital and in each of the provinces. He also indicated the need for suitable regulations to be worked out in mutual agreement with Balmis or his representative.[6]

But Balmis, who was in Caracas, acted differently, although in fact giving priority to the royal order. As stated earlier, he had learned a lesson from what he had seen in Europe, and in the experience acquired during his trip from La Coruña to Caracas. He therefore believed it was not possible to establish vaccination houses for financial reasons, nor was the utilization of hospital wards feasible for such a purpose because they were governed by their own administrations, and were limited in number and in funds.

He probably exchanged impressions with the governor and captain-general of the province, Manuel de Guevara y Vasconcelos, as well as with other individuals who had been selected to organize the work plan to be followed. In any event, it was agreed to support his decision that he was against

> the principles of depositing this precious preservative in the Hospitals, Orphanages and Foundling Homes, because, in addition to the dislike and ennui with which these establishments are usually regarded, which contributes considerably to turning the public away, it is also turned away by the lack of cleanliness and the weak and sickly constitution of their inmates; so the mothers do not want to have their children vaccinated, except the healthiest and strongest children, according to what I have seen everywhere.

The reply of the governor of the island of Margarita, addressed to the Most Excellent Don José Antonio Caballero, minister of grace and justice, on 22 December 1804 justified the impossibility of complying with the royal order, as there were neither funds nor a hospital for the troops, nor "a capable physician to perform the innoculations."[7] In summary, no vaccination house could be set up in Caracas nor could a hospital ward be equipped for that purpose.

On the other hand, on 15 April, toward the end of the first month of Balmis's stay in the country, he formally proposed to the governor and captain-general that a Central Vaccination Board be set up under the authority of the government, which would direct all matters related to the vaccine in the region. In this proposal Balmis was as explicit as he was objective, covering practically all the important points. It was such a perfect document that the same comment could be made about it as was made by Aníbal Ruiz Moreno regarding the rules given by Balmis to Salvany when the expedition was subdivided in La Guaira: "These instructions are outstanding for their foresight, scientific eagerness, tact and organizational spirit. It is an excellent proof of the capability of the individual who drew them up."

Balmis's proposals consisted of items which, in summary, expressed the following views:[8]

• Integrate the Central Vaccination Board. It should be made up of the highest civil and religious authorities in their capacity as protectors; some of the most prominent citizens; an equal number of physicians; and, as voting members, the mayor and the attorney-general of the municipal government.

• Create a secretariat and specify the duties of the two secretaries, one administrative and the other technical.

• State the objectives of the weekly meetings.

• Consider the advisability of an appropriate place for the meetings, as well as for the administration of the vaccinations. Plan measures for the eradication of smallpox.

• Appoint two physicians to be responsible for the vaccinations in alternate months; provide free services to the public.

• All members of the board should serve in an honorary capacity; only the physicians responsible for giving the vaccinations should receive payment when funds are available.

• Prohibit vaccination without prior written permission from the board.

• Provide constant information to the authorities; request the bishops to ask parochial priests to send lists of births in their districts.

- Make provision in the event of smallpox epidemics to send out a medical vaccinator, to be paid from governmental funds of the affected locality.
- Appoint investigators to carry out research on cowpox.
- Study the effects of vaccination on other diseases, particularly on yellow fever and the plague.[9]
- The technical secretary should record possible discoveries and immediately notify the director of the expedition, whose duty it is to insert such information in his logbook.

The governor studied the proposals and approved them on 23 April. After a preliminary conference held in his residence, where the main items contained in the proposals were discussed, particularly that regarding the integration of the board, invitations were sent out and the date was set for the first formal meeting.

Balmis's original recommendations received unanimous support, with only slight modifications designed to clarify certain points in accordance with local experience and circumstances, as follows:[10]

- The board should consist of ten lay ecclesiastical members, seven professors of medicine and surgery, and two secretaries, one of whom should be a physician; all should be under the sponsorship of the provincial authorities.
- "One out of every four children who are born every day in the city" should be vaccinated in the houses designated. The vaccination fluid should be sent to those places where necessary, and measures should be adopted to maintain those establishments.
- At the weekly meetings each secretary should present relevant observations in his respective field to the captain-general and to the bishop and report on "situations and news in the information whereof they might be interested."
- Two physicians responsible for the vaccinations should be appointed each month so "there will be constantly two who shall alternate by months. . ."

If it seems odd that no reference was made to arm-to-arm vaccination, it should be remembered that this practice had been categorically prohibited by a proclamation of 5 April by the governor and captain-general, which was announced in the most important towns.[11]

Although it may be self-evident, the heterogeneous composition of the board had a deliberate purpose: to assemble the most outstanding personalities in the government, the community, and the medical guild.

The installation of the Central Vaccination Board took place, with all solemnity, on 28 April 1804.

The governor and captain-general, the archbishop of the diocese, the quartermasters of the army and the Royal Treasury, and the regent of the Royal Court were declared protectors. Other members included the mayor and the attorney-general of the municipal government, as voting members; the Count of San Javier, Francisco Javier Ustáriz; Manuel Fierro; Ignacio Canibell; Luis Rivas; two priests; and José Antonio Montenegro and J. I. Moreno. The physicians were Felipe Tamariz, José Domingo Díaz, José Joaquín Hernández, Lorenzo Lasa, Vicente Salias, Santiago Limardo, and José Justo Arnanda. As scientific and political secretaries, Díaz and Gabriel Ponte were designated, respectively. Aranda was appointed custodian and distributor of the fluid; Díaz and Limardo were to select those who would be in charge of the vaccination in Caracas and other cities and towns of the province.

It should be noted that Tamariz and Limardo were the first to be appointed vaccination directors, but both excused themselves—Tamariz on account of poor eyesight, and Limardo because of his daily duties at the Charity Hospital. Aranda, who volunteered,[12] was accepted, to be assisted by Salias.

Since the original objective called for two physicians to administer the public vaccinations, the chief physician was requested to make the respective appointments; this did not occur, however, and Aranda remained as the sole official vaccinator.

At the installation ceremony it was agreed to hold subsequent meetings at the residence of the Count of San Javier[13] every Sunday from 11 A.M. to noon and, temporarily, to give public vaccinations during the same hour. Shortly afterwards the schedule was changed, and the meetings were held every Saturday at 5 P.M. Futhermore, approval was given to pay the expenses of the secretariat, a concierge, and other minor costs from city funds upon submission of an account by the secretary and approval by the Royal Court.[14]

During its entire existence, the board functioned as a mixed body with the same membership, except for the changes in its participants that took place as a consequence of the reorganization of 1807, which will be described later under the heading, Second Stage: 1807-08. All its meetings were presided over by the governor and captain-general.

Initial Activities

The first decisions concerned the appointment of several committees. One was to draft a report on "how to assure the legitimacy and perpetuity" of the vaccine fluid in the capital and its provinces; the members of this committee were Montenegro, Ustáriz, and Salias.

Another committee was designed to advise on valid procedures for the dissemination of the vaccine "so it would not degenerate and it would be possible to achieve the total destruction of the natural smallpox"; its members were the two physicians, Díaz and Limardo, and Canibell.

A third committee, appointed to prepare a plan "to extinguish soon and efficiently the natural smallpox contagion in the Capital and other places of the Province," consisted of Tamariz, Moreno, and Hernández.

Díaz and Salias were requested to write concise instructions to be circulated for the purpose of helping the medical men and other individuals who were going to give the inoculations

> to know and distinguish the true and the false vaccine; the good results of the former and the harmful of the latter; the nature of the pustules; the condition of the substance and how to apply it usefully; and observations to be made depending on the diversity of the condition of the vaccine; and when and why the fluid is fast or slow in reaching maturity, etc.

Each one of these committees complied immediately with its obligations; the governor and captain-general submitted a report for the consideration of the archbishop and the members of the board, and at a meeting on 26 May—after the departure of the Balmis Expedition—he read his personal report on the perpetuity and dissemination of the fluid. By the end of the month the board was able to express its opinion on two basic items that concerned it most: 1) the indefinite preservation of the vaccine fluid; and 2) its dissemination to the other population centers of the country.

The impossibility of dispatching the vaccine to the provinces was recognized, and it was agreed that Caracas should become the permanent repository of the vaccine, from whence it would be sent to the provinces when necessary. Furthermore, it was agreed that its preservation should be the direct responsibility of the medical director of vaccinations who, in the absence of a special place to store it, should keep it in his own home. Thus Aranda performed the vaccinations in his own home at nine-day intervals. (We point this out because during the second stage of the board Governor Juan de las Casas referred to "the weekly vaccinations.")

From the beginning the people's distrust of the new method had to be alleviated, while, on the other hand, precautions had to be taken to avoid the possible spread of false vaccine. For this purpose the approved program was formally initiated during the board's first month of activity, when the governor and captain-general sent an announcement to the lieutenants and chief justices requesting them to prevent, in their jurisdictions, the administration of vaccination by inexperienced individuals—this caused some protests. These instructions were then reinforced by ratifying what was already categorically prohibited, that is, the continued use of "variolization" (inoculation with the smallpox virus), since this outdated and dangerous procedure had been replaced by the harmless arm-to-arm innoculation of vaccination fluid.

On 14 June the governor, through Ponte, his administrative secretary, sent another circular to all provincial authorities advising them of the foundation and objectives of the Central Vaccination Board, its working arrangements, and the cooperation expected, insisting among other things on the need to vaccinate all newborn infants.

Persuasive and Coercive Measures

Although there was general receptivity, apprehension and reluctance on the part of the public are the obstacles that vaccination has had to face from the date of its discovery to the present time. It should therefore not seem strange that during the period under discussion difficulties arose in Caracas and in the villages in the interior of the province where, for example, an unusual case of *tucupido* was recorded. The people's revulsion and fear of this disease reached such extremes that they fled the area; when the vaccinator from Guanare made his appearance nobody showed up.

Such apprehension was also apparent among the Indians, according to a communication from the governor of Guayana and Father Buenaventura de San Celedonio, prefect of the missions of the Catalonian Capuchins, which was read at the board's meeting of 12 October 1805. The Indians in Sanare fled because of their fear of the vaccine.

The coercive measures that were applied were therefore sometimes justified. In Caracas, following a proposal by the regent of the Royal Court, it was decreed on 11 August 1804 that the mayors of all boroughs should find out who had not had smallpox vaccine in their respective districts in order to summon them to receive it. On the same date it was decided that the governor and captain-general should arouse public opinion through a proclamation.

This was done on 20 August, and four copies of the statement were placed at central locations in the city. According to the text, children were summoned to receive the vaccine fluid and should appear promptly at the place designated for that purpose at the time and on the day indicated, under penalty of a fine of 25 pesos,

> which will be incurred by those who are in a position to pay this fine; the parents and other people in charge of those summoned who fail to appear without cause will be subject to the same fine as those who, without proper license, inoculate the vaccine outside the designated house and time; they will be punished by nine days in prison or an equal amount of time in public

works, depending on the transgressors, upon whom, because of lack of property, this monetary fine cannot be imposed.

On 13 April 1805 a new proclamation was published to encourage unprotected citizens to receive vaccinations. A complaint received from Guanare stated that the residents refused to be vaccinated, whereupon the governor and captain-general proposed, with the approval of the board, to punish them with ten days in prison.

Such coercive measures were used only occasionally, however, and were not applied systematically; on the contrary, the archbishop's cooperation was frequently requested as he was a fervent advocate of vaccinations. He was asked to approach the parish priests and urge them to apply all the persuasive means within their power to cope with the scruples and difficulties as they arose.

In this author's earlier publication, *The Balmis Expedition in Venezuela*,[15] we confirmed Lanning's opinion of the intuition of the chamber physician, José Felipe Flores—the glory of Guatemalan medicine—for having insisted on the importance of the pulpit in creating a proper climate for the vaccination program, as well as the undeniable fact that Balmis's tremendous success in Caracas, Bogotá, and elsewhere may very well be attributed to the unrestricted support he received from both civil and church authorities.

In responding to a report of the chief justice of Río del Tocuyo, in which he discussed the villagers' refusal to accept the benefits of the vaccine, it was agreed

> that he try to overcome that resistance with gentle means, based on his knowledge of the nature of the villagers, and that only in the event that he could not overcome their resistance by such means should he resort to the application of slight penalties, such as one or two days of imprisonment for the most rebellious.

A unique incident was reported by the lieutenant chief justice of Carora: some ladies refused to go to the vaccinator's house, "because they felt the high privileges of their nobility were being slighted." In view of this situation the board resolved that the vaccinator should give home service, but that he should ask said ladies to pay a fee for this privilege.

Conservation of the Vaccination Fluid

In the same manner as the service performed by Aranda at the level of the Central Board, responsibility for the conservation of the vaccine was vested in local vaccinators who were trained for this task. They were to make sure that the pustules of those vaccinated were not lost; make the mothers keep the appointments; and be guided in their work by the biweekly list of baptized children sent in by the parish priests. As had been foreseen, it was of course very difficult to achieve such objectives in the interior of the country due to the lack of physicians, the low density rate of the people, and their poor economic resources; all these factors contributed to problems of communication.

Very frequently, therefore, the vaccine was lost, and consequently it became necessary to obtain more of it from Caracas or the closest city. On the other hand, it was always possible to conserve the fluid in the capital, at least during the tenure of the Central Board, and even during the period when it became paralyzed. This is a praiseworthy feat that may be attributed to the zeal and activity displayed by the official custodian and distributor of the fluid, the surgeon José Justo Aranda.

Efforts in favor of conserving the fluid were also carried out without having to resort to arm-to-arm inoculations, and on 2 June 1804 Limardo and Montenegro were commissioned to write a complete report on the subject. They complied partially. At the next meeting on 9 June they were authorized to carry out experiments that would lead to the achievement of this purpose. At the meeting on 28 July, Rivas, a member of the board, read a paper he had received explaining how to conserve the vaccine virus by means of reducing pustulous scabs to powder.

At a meeting on 6 October the president produced a translated letter from a Dr. Lascalis on the nature and properties of the vaccination scab, along with four printed treatises on the subject and a box containing the vaccination fluid in the form of scabs, all of which had been brought from Philadelphia by Dr. Luis López Méndez. Contrary to what had been expected, the inoculations with this substance proved to be negative. Limardo was thereupon instructed to

> collect and keep the fluid for nine, ten, and even twelve days, as well as the scabs of pustules, in glasses covered with vellum or English taffeta at their junctures, and to submit both, after keeping them for the time deemed necessary to the experiment, and the results desired to be achieved with these operations, because of the negative effect of those delivered by Don Luis López Méndez, which had been brought from the Anglo-American institutions.

In addition, some time later a letter from Governor Inciarte of Guayana stated that the vaccination fluid sent by the governor of Cumaná had been spoiled twice—no doubt because of the distance between these cities and the excessive heat. He had not been able to get another supply because there was no more in Aragua or in the province of Barinas. By a royal order of 6 September 1805, Inciarte was instructed to try to obtain good vaccination scabs in Caracas or some other nearby province which, if pulverized and dissolved in water with the point of a surgical lancet, would produce the same effect. Apparently, as with López Méndez's material, the experience of Limardo, Montenegro, and Inciarte had negative results, as arm-to-arm inoculations continued to be performed for a long time.[16]

Distribution of the Vaccine

If the concern about conserving the vaccination fluid was legitimate, so was the board's effort to gradually extend the benefits of the vaccine to as many locations as possible, simultaneously exercising "control" in order to achieve the established objectives.

The procedure adopted for distribution consisted in asking the magistrates and lieutenant chief justices to send to Caracas

> the respective medical men and individuals with a good will and ability to learn to attend the operation and learn how to perform it, as well as to distinguish the true from the false vaccine . . . and to bring the necessary number of children or adults who, depending on the distance, would carry the vaccination fluid . . . the expense to be covered out of the funds of the respective towns, the community funds of the Indians, or private donations.[17]

In the event that no physicians or other able people were available, the board agreed to send out a medical man, provided all his expenses were paid. It should be remembered that doctors Díaz and Limardo had been instructed in Caracas to examine, teach, and *authorize* all applicants, for without such authorization they could not perform the vaccinations. In many instances, however, the board had to adapt itself to local circumstances and allow candidates from small towns to go on to other important centers nearby to receive their training and licenses.

Only in Valencia, Barinas, Puerto Cabello, and Maracaibo did physicians act as vaccinators. In the great majority of the other cities and towns private individuals underwent training and obtained their certificates. There were cases where the municipal government had to take over: the city of Barquisimeto, for example, at first paid all transportation expenses, but later, because of the vaccinator's poor financial resources, it was agreed that on his trips to neighboring towns the authorities should pay him half a *real* for each vaccinated person. In Carora the deputy mayor was appointed vaccinator.

The records show that the board reviewed each potential licensee, and that a vaccinator was not authorized until all requirements had been satisfied. In 1804 eighteen individuals were examined and received approval to vaccinate in the towns of the province. The records are very rich in details, and not only provide information about the successive appointments, but about the interesting chronological order in which the vaccination process spread over the entire country. By 1804 Maracaibo, the island of Margarita, and Guayana were covered, and by 1805 the vaccine had extended to the province of Cumaná. Table 1 shows the locations covered as of 1 February 1806.

The Indian villages under the direction of the Capuchin priests were not neglected: Guama, Chivacoa, Urachiche, and Yaritagua were assigned to the vaccinator of Barquisimeto. According to Governor Cagigal, by 22 May 1805 "the Indians vaccinated in Cumaná province amounted to 20,000."[18]

It is of interest that in February 1805 authorization was granted to Father José Félix Espinosa de los Monteros, of the village of Arenales, "to take the fluid and qualify a vaccinator in El Tocuyo to set up the vaccination in said village, which he has offered to do at his own expense."

From the beginning it was the practice to ask parish priests to submit biweekly lists of baptized children for the purpose of conserving and distributing the vaccination fluid through proper computations of the available supplies.

In the scientific secretariat headed by Díaz, monthly vaccination lists were centralized, a requirement that had been established when the board was set up. This was facilitated by reports made by the vaccinators, either through territorial judges or chief justices. The lists specified dates, ages, and other pertinent observations. At each meeting, the secretary submitted reports and commented on those items relating to vaccination techniques. For example, when Díaz reported on the difficulties experienced by the vaccinator of La Guaira, in the sense that the vaccines did not "take," probably due to the region's hot climate, the governor and captain-general proposed, and the motion seconded by the other board members, that the vaccinator be instructed to perform the inoculations in more protected parts of the body, such as the thighs.

On another occasion, because of reports of inflammation observed on the patients' arms in Villa de San Carlos, Díaz devised a method to avoid "the accidents and symptoms the vaccinated experienced there." In Villa del Calabozo, in view of repeated reports by Carlos del Pozo of the disagreeable consequences experienced due to vaccinating with the same lancet used indiscriminatingly for surgical operations, qualified vaccinators

Table I. PLACES AND NUMBER OF PEOPLE VACCINATED AS RECORDED IN THE MINUTES OF 1 FEBRUARY 1806 OF THE CENTRAL VACCINATION BOARD OF CARACAS.

Aguas de Culebra	601	Mariara	118
Araguita	501	Marin	398
Araure	748	Maiquetia	64
Arenales	733	Naiguatá	43
Barquisimeto	9,795	Ocumare	83
Baul	545	Ospino	201
Burburata	796	Paracotos	222
Cagua	16	Petare	853
Calabozo	1,012	Puerto Cabello	2,241
Caracas	3,702	Quibor	1,678
Caramacate	450	Rio del Tocuyo	147
Carayaca	116	Sanare	127
Carora	1,561	San Antonio	182
Caucagua	117	San Carlos	3,393
Chacao	117	San Diego	93
Chaguaramas	573	San Esteban	147
Choroni	699	San Felipe	1,390
Chuao	284	San José	420
Cojo	11	San Sebastian	167
Cocorote	1,288	Santa Lucia	1,597
Cojedes	591	Tacata	203
Curarigua	517	Tarmas	154
Cuyagua	104	Tinaco	1,211
Guacara	391	Tinajas	536
Guama	718	Tinaquillo	724
Guanare	540	Tiznados	780
Guarenas	1,491	Tocuyo	1,412
Guarico	109	Turmero	654
Guarire	371	Valencia	992
Guayos	176	Valle	48
Guayra	552	Valleseco	313
Guigue	171	Victoria	550
Lagunitas	732	Villa de Cura	706
Macarao	106	Yaritagua	2,321
Macuto	13	Ipire	433
Maracay	257	Total	55,105

were instructed to use the vaccination lancet exclusively for that purpose and not for other minor surgery.

In accordance with Balmis's original order, vaccinations were given as a free public service. There were exceptions, however, as in the case of the agreement with the vaccinator in Barquisimeto, and the ladies who refused to go to the home of the vaccinator in Carora. Another interesting solution found by the lieutenant of Ospino was to consolidate the vaccinations in his community, which he achieved through private contributions: one *real* was paid to the vaccinator by each white person, and half a *real* by nonwhites. Aside from these examples, the minutes of the board reveal that many vaccinators asked to be rewarded for their services; in general, when local funds were available their petitions were granted.[19]

The Board Takes General Measures

As the vaccination process advanced, many useful provisions were adopted. In June 1804 it was decreed that physician members of the board take a census in the city of individuals afflicted by natural smallpox, together with their addresses and other data; if indicated by the findings of the survey, special provisions should be undertaken to vaccinate them. Another measure, approved on 7 July of the same year, provided for the vaccination of shiploads of Negroes; this was enforced in La Guaira and Puerto Cabello.

Simultaneously, a census was taken in Caracas of all houses in which patients with smallpox had been cared for in the past. They were subject to cleansing and fumigating, as were the hospitals, including the Military Hospital. In the case of hospitals for contagious diseases, it was recommended that special wards be equipped for the isolation of smallpox patients to avoid spreading the contagion to other patients or to visitors. Numerous cases of contagion had been regularly observed, due to the common hospitalization of smallpox patients, but this was corrected thanks to the pressure of the Central Vaccination Board.

On the other hand, on 26 January 1805 it was agreed to extend to the hospitals of La Guaira and Puerto Cabello the practice of vaccinating all patients who had not had smallpox, which the General Hospital of Caracas had adopted at the end of 1804; by that time Caracas was already free of smallpox cases, except for some in the General Hospital. Upon the recommendation of the regent of the Royal Court, it was resolved that in order to hasten the fumigations Limardo be appointed commissioner of the board to carry them out, together with the general officers of the Royal Treasury.

On several occasions the board warned about the danger involved in opening graves containing the bodies of people who had died of smallpox, and urged the construction of separate graveyards in order to abolish the common practice of interments in temples. The captain-general asked the archbishop to instruct the parish priests to distinguish the graves of smallpox victims. Regarding the practice of interment in temples, on 5 January 1805 Francisco Javier Ustáriz submitted a report urging the abolition of the practice. (Apparently the habit persisted for many years, however, because in 1827 the *Libertador* issued a decree, fully ratifying the Spanish order, which provided that all bodies, without exception, be buried in graveyards, even if they were only temporary sites.)

In August 1804, His Most Illustrious Excellency Francisco de Ibarra issued precise instructions to the priests of Turmero, Cagua, and El Escovar requesting them to make lists of their parishoners and their baptismal records available to the lieutenant chief justice of the province. Over the course of time such instructions became generalized for all villages and towns of the interior.

On 1 June 1805 the governor and captain-general proposed, and the board agreed, to send out circulars to the lieutenant chief justices of the province who had not complied as yet with the order to procure the fluid and to qualify a vaccinator, reminding them to do so. At the same time they were instructed to find out from the governors and commanders of adjacent provinces the condition of their vaccine and the success obtained in their respective jurisdictions.

Finally, on 3 August, on the recommendation of Díaz, a circular was distributed among the commanders of the military forces ordering them to strictly supervise the effective vaccination of recruits and those who, in spite of previous instructions, had still not been immunized.

Priority Given to the Discovery of Cowpox

Before he departed, one of Balmis's recommendations was that the existence of cowpox or cow disease in the country should be verified, as ratified by royal order in correspondence received in September 1804.[20] Consequently, on 20 October, taking into account the vast knowledge and zeal of Carlos del Pozo, an "ingenious subject who had started to make electric machines. . . ,"[21] and who resided in Villa del Calabozo where there were great herds of cattle, the board entrusted him with this mission. Later the archbishop proposed the advisability of encouraging the discovery of cowpox by awarding a prize. This idea was accepted, although we do not know if it was carried out.

By the end of 1804 Pozo reported that he had conducted research among the cattle and that he had been able to verify the existence of cowpox through inoculations given to several individuals, who subsequently experienced all the reactions of the real vaccine. He proposed to repeat the experiments "as soon as the favorable season arrives, in order to comply better with the recommendations of the Board."[22] In recognition of the success achieved by this illustrious scientist it was resolved to appoint him immediately as a member of the board and as its correspondent in Calabozo.

Correspondence received from Pozo in January 1805 furnished data about the nature and properties of the vaccination pustules in the plains of Calabozo. Thereupon he was instructed to request the chief justice of the town to attest to the authenticity of the vaccine. He was also asked for a detailed report on the keloids that were observed on four vaccinated individuals after the scab of the pustule had fallen off.

Our character Pozo proved to be very active. In August 1805 the members of the board learned that he had discovered cowpox pustules in the cows; he promised to make a more detailed report of this discovery later. The following is recorded in the board's minutes of 26 October:

> Don Carlos del Pozo introduced a twenty-one-year-old darky by the name of Casildo Herrera, whom he had vaccinated in Villa del Calabozo with fluid taken from the cows. He gave an exact account of everything he had observed during the course of his pustules, which coincided with statements in his previous reports. The individual, who had been vaccinated on the 14th, was examined by the Board, and the evidence of Don Carlos del Pozo's statement was found and verified. Nothing else could be observed, due to the dessication of the pustules, other than their larger size than that of those vaccinated arm-to-arm.

Here it should be mentioned that in a letter from Balmis of 4 February 1805, received in Venezuela in July, he stated that he and some others had discovered the cowpox in several places in Mexico, including Valladolid, Michoacán, and Puebla. This news was transmitted to Pozo. The report to Charles IV informing him in detail about the discovery of cowpox in Venezuela received the approval of the Higher Medicine Board of Madrid, which praised the activity and zeal of the Central Vaccination Board in Caracas. The *Gaceta de Madrid* (Madrid Gazette) of 14 October 1806 published an account of the discoveries made in Mexico as well as in Calabozo.

Supporters of the Board

In the first part of our study dealing with the arrival of the expedition in Venezuela,[23] we pointed out the liberal attitude of the governor and captain-general, Manuel Guevara y Vasconcelos: not only did he receive Balmis most enthusiastically, but he offered him all kinds of help. He was indeed proud of the expedition, and he extended his strong support to the Central Vaccination Board as long as he held his high political investiture, which he did until his death on 9 October 1807.

Guevara y Vasconcelos could have limited his assistance to mere acquiescence to the draft of the board's plan as proposed by Balmis, and to support of its operation for a very limited period. But, contrary to other representatives of the crown with whom Balmis dealt, Guevara y Vasconcelos became a permanent protector of the board, to such an extent that he never failed to attend a single meeting. More significant, as chairman of the board he took an active part in the discussions—even in the scientific details—and in the resolutions, as well as in many of the initiatives that were taken. Had it not been for his effective participation the Vaccination Board would probably have failed, or at least it would not have achieved such great success.

Obviously there were times when the cooperation of the church was imperative. Hence, within his sphere of influence, the contributions of Archbishop Francisco de Ibarra (who died in September 1806) and his successor were most decisive factors. Thanks to the leadership of these high prelates the activities of the clergy were very effective, particularly in disseminating information, which was so necessary for the acceptance of the vaccine by the public. Of great use, also, was the compliance of parish priests in providing lists of baptized children for the purpose of spreading the vaccination.

Sometimes people's apprehensions are strange and inexplicable, and it happened that, in the village of San José de Tiznados, word was spread that the vaccination fluid had been introduced by enemies of the state, perhaps for the purpose of creating an unfavorable atmosphere for the government. This incident caused the lieutenant chief justice of that locality to issue a proclamation denying the story, and Guevara y Vasconcelos gave orders that the statement should be published. In summary, all possible efforts were made to vaccinate all citizens, and for this purpose orders were given to post the proclamation at the most frequented locations so that it would be seen by everybody.

The physicians performed their duties satisfactorily, but undoubtedly the most outstanding figures in the initial smallpox vaccination campaign carried out by the Central Vaccination Board were José Domingo Díaz and José Justo Aranda.

Díaz was both the scientific secretary of the board and the trainer and examiner of the vaccinators who came to Caracas. He was the first to try to locate the cowpox, and used every opportunity to emphasize the importance of the vaccine and to sway public opinion in its favor. His statistical tables and numerous instructions and memoirs make it easier for us today to understand the historical development of the vaccination campaign in Venezuela. The statistics are indeed excellent, considering that at that time this field was not yet at the peak it later acquired in the medical sciences—his accuracy even included calculations of the daily average of the births in the parishes of Caracas between 1796 and 1803.

In brief, Díaz's name is so closely linked to the Central Vaccination Board that he was its major motivator during its first stage—a true champion of the vaccine. His concept of the issue was so complete that he contributed the greatest number of writings to the incipient bibliography on smallpox and vaccine; some of his reports predate the arrival of Balmis. With justification, in October 1805 the board awarded him a vote of confidence.

Díaz is better known in the history of his country for his political activities, however, for he epitomized the most resentful hatred of Bolívar and the cause of the emancipative revolution. Precisely the reverse of that aspect of his personality was his scientific attitude, particularly his extraordinary early work in the field of sanitation. Venezuelan historians will continue, with reason, to criticize this fanatical enemy of the father of the country, the author of *Recuerdos sobre la Rebelión de Caracas*, but, as we have asserted elsewhere,[24] medical historians, bound by the strictest impartiality, cannot but recognize his true professional merits.

The surgeon Aranda was from the beginning entrusted with the conservation and distribution of the vaccination fluid, and this responsibility was of extraordinary value. Thanks to his zealous activities the vaccination fluid was preserved in Caracas during the crisis suffered by the Vaccination Board in 1806-07. During its reorganization in November 1807, Governor and Captain-General Juan de las Casas, Guevara y Vasconcelos's successor, reported that the vaccination fluid was being conserved without any interruption in public vaccinations, which were being administered in Aranda's home.

Chart prepared by José Domingo Díaz of the people vaccinated in various towns in Venezuela. Caracas, 12 March 1805.

Numerical Balance

In the long run the numerical language is the most convincing. Thus, in order to appraise the exact dimensions of the task performed, let us begin by stating that, according to Díaz, by the end of 1804 some 25,000 people had been vaccinated in fifty-one cities and towns. By 31 July 1805 the figure for the entire country had reached 30,804 people of all ages. In February 1806, one year and ten months after the Central Vaccination Board had been set up, its activities had spread to seventy-one localities, including the capital, and the vaccinated amounted to a total of 55,105 (Table 1).[25]. Four years after the departure of the Royal Expedition, according to the *Gaceta de Caracas* of 3 December 1817, "from March 28, 1804 to the same day in 1808, 104,700 people were vaccinated in this province."[26]

It is not up to us to presume to make comparisons with other places included in Balmis's triumphant tour, but we do believe that when all figures are available and treated statistically, the record achieved in Venezuela will be in the forefront. In synthesis, Venezuelan epidemiologists should feel satisfied with the scope of our first massive antismallpox campaign.

A significant detail is the incidence of smallpox at the beginning of the vaccinations, particularly in Caracas, where the disease showed a high degree of morbidity. During the first year, 1804, isolated cases were observed, especially in the General Hospital. From 1805 on, the most frequent observation in the records, sometimes almost like a refrain, is that the doctors of the board reported that no cases of smallpox existed in the city. Only in 1808 did a severe epidemic occur in Cumaná, according to a communication from the chief of that province to the Central Vaccination Board. Until 1810, the period to which this narration refers, no other serious epidemic of the disease was recorded.

Bibliographic Balance

The introduction of antismallpox vaccine gave rise simultaneously to the first Venezuelan bibliography on the subject. Several important papers were prepared at that time by Díaz, Tamariz, Hernández, Limardo, Salias, Antonio Gómez and others. Some were produced during Balmis's stay in Venezuela, but the majority were submitted to the Central Vaccination Board or read at its meetings. Most likely those papers played some part in the success of the board. Be that as it may, all of them were of course in manuscript form, because the printing press did not come to Venezuela until 1808. Had it arrived earlier we would have today medical reprints dating from the end of the eighteenth centuty.

Unfortunately, the contents of the Venezuelan medical bibliography must be rescued gradually. It represents a wide range of research, full of intense interest to our bibliographers and historians. By looking at the titles it is evident that the author who made the most contributions was Díaz,[27] followed by Salias and others.[28]

The Activities Are Interrupted

The final activities of the Central Vaccination Board, acccording to the records of the first stage, took place during the first months of 1806. At its last meetings Díaz presented and justified his statistical work, which showed the number of persons who had survived because of the antismallpox immunization program.

The board met regularly until the peace of the colony was upset by General Francisco de Miranda's unsuccessful invasions in April and August of 1806. At that time its operations collapsed, and there is therefore a gap in its Book of Resolutions from 8 March 1806 to 16 November 1807.

The government's attention was concentrated exclusively on political events. Due to grave developments at the beginning of 1806 the board's meetings were interrupted, Andrés Bello wrote later, in the first of the minutes he was to write in his capacity as secretary after the board was reorganized.

With a break in the continuity of the availability of the vaccine fluid, it could not be transported to most of the villages in the interior of the province; this is turn had repercussions in the sense that the prejudice against preventive procedures was strengthened.

SECOND STAGE: 1807–08

Reorganization of the Board

The twenty-month paralysis of a scientific body may not seem extraordinary, but if one takes into account that, simultaneously, the political history of Venezuela was reaching the much-longed-for climax of independence, it is understandable that any prospect of change would have had a serious influence on the country's stability. Moreover, there existed the grave threat of military invasions of the style of those conducted by General Miranda, which deeply shook the foundations of the government Shortly thereafter, in the key two-year period, 1810-11, the emancipative revolution broke out, an event that explains the curtailed activities of the board upon the reassumption of its functions.

In the meantime, during the board's period of inactivity its two illustrious advocates had died: Guevara y Vasconselos on 9 October 1807, and Ibarra on 19 September 1806.

On 26 October 1807 the Municipal Council of Caracas became impatient and sent a petition to the acting governor urging him to reinstate the board, primarily because they feared the vaccine fluid would be lost.

Colonel Juan de las Casas, in his capacity as royal lieutenant and war auditor, had assumed military and political command of the province of Venezuela. He eventually offered the excuse that he had only postponed action on the petition for the necessary period of time needed to take over the complicated matters of the captaincy-general. In any event, he heeded the petition, and the second stage of the Central Vaccination Board took place on 16 November 1807 in the home of the Count of San Javier, which had served as headquarters for previous meetings.[29]

De las Casas, as the new governor and captain-general and chairman of the Central Board, informed about the circumstances that had interrupted its activities, resolved that the weekly meetings should be resumed. He introduced some changes in the Board of Directors: Joaquín de Mosquera y Figueroa, acting regent, replaced Councilman Antonio López Quintana, who had been promoted to the Supreme Council of the Indies; Father Alejandro Echezuría filled the vacancy left by the death of Moreno; the physicians José Antonio Alamo, Francisco Isnardi, and José Antonio Gómez replaced Díaz and Aranda, who were sick at that time; and Andrés Bello[30] substituted for Ponte, who was away from the city. Gómez and Bello assumed, respectively, the medical and political secretariats. At a meeting on 28 November, upon a motion by Canibell, the chief accountant, it was resolved to consider Isnardi and Alamo, as well as the acting secretaries, as members of the board, and they were requested to nominate substitutes should they be absent or ill. (Ponte resigned formally from the political secretariat on 1 March 1808.) Aranda continued as vaccination director.

At the reorganization meeting the chairman informed the group that, in spite of the serious problems that had arisen, the vaccine fluid had been conserved thanks to the weekly vaccinations that had continued to be given in Aranda's home. On the other hand, after inquiring about the present situation, they learned there were no cases of smallpox in the hospitals and only one in the district of San Pablo. At the next meeting on 9 December this case could not be confirmed, and all present agreed that Caracas was free of smallpox at the time.

A few months later de las Casas deemed it advisable to advise the authorities in Spain about the status of the vaccine in the provinces; the reorganization of the Central Board; the resolutions put forth at its meeting; and the need for the king to propose new regulations to improve some aspects of the board's operation. De las Casas's report to the Spanish minister of grace and justice on 26 March 1808[31] pointed out that the vaccination campaign had been interrupted for several reasons, among them the invasion attempts of Miranda; the fact that almost the entire province was under arms; the doubts of the public, which could never be completely allayed; the total absence of medical personnel in the remote villages; and the lack of any remuneration for the vaccinators. The king, by a royal order of 3 August 1807, gave instructions to convey his most affectionate appreciation to all individuals on the board for their zeal, disinterest in personal gain, and efficiency.

Work Program

As a consequence of the circumstances that resulted in the involuntary interruption of the board's functions, and in view of the reports submitted respectively by Ustáriz and Díaz, the work of the reorganized board centered around two basic points: the conservation of vaccine fluid, and its distribution to the largest possible number of people and localities. Certain measures were employed to achieve these objectives.

In support of the first point, at the suggestion of Díaz, who largely blamed the indolence of some lieutenant justices for the loss of the fluid, it was resolved to include a clause in the entitlements of the lieutenants that made them responsible for conserving the fluid, and request them to render an account thereof upon the expiration of their terms of office.

Several resolutions were taken on the second point: records to be kept of children to be vaccinated; educational campaigns; and compensation for the vaccinators.

To the system of monthly lists of the vaccinated sent in by all the parties was added a requirement making it compulsory that these lists be accompanied by records made out by the clergy who performed baptisms in each parish, for the purpose of making it easier for the board to compare them and take necessary corrective measures; furthermore they had to submit lists of the babies who died before being vaccinated. Incidentally, the lists of the baptized continued after the installation of the Republic.

With regard to educational measures, the vicar general was instructed to urge parish priests to give persuasive and educational sermons in order to revive the public's confidence in the vaccine; compulsory measures would be a last resort. As for the advisability of compensation for the vaccinators, it was agreed that subordinate vaccination boards should seek ways to pay them;[32] to that end the possibility was suggested that the families of those who were vaccinated make a contribution, even if it were only a modest amount.

The most important decision was taken on 19 December 1807, however, thanks to a proposal by Luis de Rivas; its purpose was to consolidate the most successful efforts to reestablish vaccinations in the villages of the interior. The creation of subordinate boards to the Central Board was approved, with the stipulation that they should be set up in the major cities of the province, and that each be made up of the lieutenant chief justice, the priest, the mayor, the attorney general, and a proportionate number of the most important citizens. Bello was the drafter of these rules and regulations, which were examined by a physician, Montenegro, and Rivas, who introduced some additions and changes. In view of these developments, and in accordance with the wishes of the board, Chairman de las Casas, decided "to send out the circular forthwith to the capital lieutenantships and commanders of the province."[33]

As with the first stage, this time all necessary steps were taken in connection with the progress of the vaccinations, so that as of December 1807 evidence existed of the required measures having been discussed and approved in Puerto Cabello, Curiepe, La Guaira, Valencia, Sabana de Ocumare, Barquisimeto, El Tocuyo Carlos, Guarenas, Turmero, Cagua, Santa Cruz, San José de la Sabana, Caruao, Macuto, Chuspa, Naiguatá, Caraballeda, Chacao, Los Teques, Petare, and Ocumare.

A justifiable resolution we cannot fail to mention was the appointment to the board of honorary members on 19 December in recognition of their important services in the vaccination effort. Such designations were made to Lieutenant-Colonel Julián de Izquierdo of Coro and the priest of Arenales, José Félix Espinosa de los Monteros.

Andrés Bello

It is important to emphasize the active role played by Andrés Bello in the activities of the Central Vaccination Board during its second and final stage. We pointed this out in 1956 in *Historia de la Sanidad en Venezuela*,[34] when we said that this was a little-known aspect of his biography. As a result, Pedro Grases, in his capacity as a member of the Editorial Commission of the *Obras Completas de Andrés Bello*, after obtaining all the information we could furnish him, investigated the matter in more depth. Subsequently an appendix to volume XX of the *Obras* appeared concerning the activities of this illustrious Venezuelan.[35] Thanks to this accurate and excellent edition, therefore, this aspect of the 1799 graduate of medicine of the Royal Pontifical University is now well known; he later became a prominent humanist in the Americas.

All the minutes of the board from 16 November 1807 to 9 April 1808 bear his signature, and they are distinguished by a neatness of style so typical of this eminent Venezuelan; sometimes they contain his personal opinions, as, for example, in those of 9 January 1808, when he pointed out the need for the civil division to make provision for the establishment of vaccinations in the villages attached to the municipal government of Caracas.

It is significant that Bello was asked to edit the regulations to create and operate the subordinate boards; he completed the task on 12 December 1807. The aforementioned appendix to the *Obras Completas* states that they must have been approved because, in a meeting of 16 January 1808, it was resolved that Gómez, as the scientific secretary, should write a summary to be sent to the interior of the country; as stated earlier, Governor de las Casas decided that when the draft was submitted all the provincial authorities should be informed about its contents by means of a circular. The regulations that served to create, organize, and outline the duties of the subordinate vaccination boards remained unpublished until 1881, when, on the occasion of the 100th anniversary of Bello's birth, the journal *Unión Médica* reproduced the entire text;[36] thereafter they were cast into oblivion until we called attention to them.[37]

In summary, in addition to his specific duties as political secretary of the board, Bello[38] was the author of other important contributions such as the aforementioned regulations and the Excise Tax Plan, which he was requested to prepare during the board's meeting of 20 February 1808. The latter was designed to establish means to finance the expenses of both secretariats, and it was praised by Díaz, Rivas, and Montenegro, a former teacher of Bello's; Rivas and Montenegro had been appointed by the board to study the merits of the plan.

Last Activities of José Domingo Díaz

José Domingo Díaz, the acting secretary, did not resume his post. The reason may be attributed to his political ideology, which was so deeply linked to the royalist cause that eventually he became a major enemy of the

Libertador and of the emancipation movement; to a serious illness from which he suffered; and, particularly, to a longstanding disagreement he had with the municipal government of Caracas, which resulted in his dismissal from his position as physician to the municipality; which in turn gave rise to a long and turbulent trial. Be that as it may, he did nominally at least retain his original appointment as scientific secretary.

During the session of 28 November 1807, only twelve days after the board was reinstated, Díaz gave a report on the period during which it had been inactive; it was of extraordinary interest and importance. Without the slightest show of fear, and backed by his considerable knowledge of the local problems of vaccination, Díaz resolutely offered concrete solutions that brought about a revision of the program. According to his report, it was quite clear that while the process of vaccination had not suffered any setbacks in the capital, in the rest of the province it had been kept up only in Coro and La Guaira; in all the other cities and towns the fluid had been lost. In his opinion this was due to three incriminating factors: 1) the ignorance and vanity of the public; 2) the indolence of the lieutenant justices; and 3) the meager remuneration of the vaccinators.

Díaz proposed three corrective measures: an intensification of the educational work carried out by the parish priests; a requirement that the lieutenants be responsible for the loss of the fluid; and fair pay for the vaccinators, either from public funds or from voluntary contributions. He also insisted on the urgency of finding the funds to cover the ordinary and necessary expenses of the board.

The final reference to Díaz is to be found in the record of the session of 15 March 1808, at which a communication of his was read. He bade the board farewell, as he would soon be leaving for Europe; asked that all reports he had filed with the Political Secretariat be forwarded to him; and turned over the archives for which he had been responsible. He in turn was asked to write a complete report of the activities of the board and of the process of vaccination since the end of 1805, a request he met with a comprehensive statement submitted on 21 March.

Having lost the protection he had enjoyed under the late Governor Guevara y Vasconcelos, and having been dismissed from his post as municipal physician, Díaz left for Spain on 9 April to try to obtain a repeal of the drastic measure taken by the council.

Governor de las Casas, who was also having troubles with the board, wished to benefit from Díaz's visit and requested the board to commission him to personally deliver a number of petitions to the Royal Court; these were to be carried by hand and to be saved in the event the ship was captured.

The governor also requested Díaz to write a history of vaccination in the province. In reality this task was the responsibility of Bello, the administrative secretary, who, as is recorded in the proceedings of the 15 March meeting, registered an energetic protest against Díaz writing such a report. It was resolved by the governor and the board that Bello should write that part of the history having to do with the economic and governmental sides, and that Díaz should do the same for the medical side.

In his final address to the board Díaz declared that

> having to go to the kingdom of Spain in search of health in other climes, I believe it my obligation to declare before this honorable body, before my departure, my gratitude and acknowledgement for the appreciation that has been shown for my services during the long time that I have been secretary; also calling attention, among other things, to the fact that I am leaving while still enjoying the post with which I have been honored, namely, that of scientific secretary; and hoping that my services in this field increase, either while living at the Court of Madrid or in whatever country in the universe that my fortune may take me to . . . .[39]

Difficulties Arise; Activities Languish; and the Board Is Terminated

Its activities had barely been resumed when the board faced a complaint brought by one of its members, the physician Salias, due to the fact that the board had resolved to replace the ailing Aranda temporarily with the surgeon Carlos Arvelo. Salias had anticipated that he would be appointed, but Aranda argued that Arvelo's appointment had become necessary due to Salias's repeated absences, and that he had acted under the authority of the late Guevara y Vasconcelos.

On 5 December 1807 Salias presented himself to claim the post, stating that his absences were due to his having to substitute for Aranda, who had not advised him of the days for vaccination. Salias claimed to possess several documents and testimonials of his good conduct, which we would present if it were deemed necessary, and that to be stripped of the commission would be a great affront to him.

Governor de las Casas ordered Aranda to submit a detailed report in order to assess the situation; after studying the report he ordered Aranda to continue as the principal person in charge of and responsible for the pus vaccine;[40] decreed that Arvelo should substitute for him during his absences or illnesses; and that Salias should not be dismissed. Thus the agreements made by the board in its session of 2 June 1804 were left in force.

Serious financial problems then arose, which Díaz had already mentioned in his first report to the reorganized board. In accordance with that statement, expenses must not exceed 400 to 500 pesos annually, and, in consideration of the benefits derived from the conservation of the vaccination fluid, this amount should be drawn from the public funds of the cities of the province and from the treasuries of the Indian villages, which should contribute a percentage of their annual income. If such contributions should exceed the amount specified, the balance could be applied to the pay of vaccinators in those places where remunerations were too low, or to other purposes the board might stipulate.

It seems that difficulties were encountered because, through legal channels, the governor had asked the king to decree by royal order that the municipal government of the capital should pay the amount due the board. During the last sessions of January 1808 it was brought to the board's attention that the municipal government flatly refused to pay from its treasury the expenses incurred by the secretariats. A month later came a letter from the High Court in Madrid indicating its refusal to approve payment of the expenses from public funds.

Of all the problems that kept arising the critical one was the serious deadlock brought about by Salias, who presented a controversial paper entitled "Reflections on the False Vaccine" at the session of 20 February 1808. The essential issue was that, based on observations of a number—a very small number in fact—of false vaccinations reported, Salias generalized to the entire population, and warned that people who had been in contact with those who had been falsely vaccinated might themselves contract smallpox. Salias concluded by proposing that all persons so exposed should go to his home six days after vaccination in order that observations concerning their safety could be made.

Governor de las Casas consulted with the other medical members of the board, and a variety of opinions were offered, all more or less in opposition to the proposal. The governor ordered those who had had false vaccinations to have a second vaccination, and requested that all experiments necessary to clear up the doubts raised by Salias should be performed. The governor especially desired Aranda to study Salias's paper, but the latter rejected this as unbecoming treatment of a university-trained doctor and prosecutor in the Medical Court. Thus, instead of provoking true scientific interest, the article resulted in a political commotion, rumors of personal intrigue, and even speculation about the reappearance of smallpox—all of which hurt the colonial authorities.

There ensued a violent disagreement between Salias and the governor,[41] who reacted in a completely unprecedented manner. Based apparently on the notion that Salias had exceeded himself in his defense and had shown a lack of respect toward both the administration and Aranda, the governor ordered that a condemnation of Salias be written into the Book of Decrees, stating that his scientific reasoning was absolutely irregular and unacceptable, and judging his intervention in the case offensive to the dignity of the board. He reprimanded Salias severely, warning him he would be ousted from the board should another such incident occur, and specifying that measures be taken to prevent such a repetition by other members of the board.

Salias, on his part, sent a lengthy appeal to the minister of grace and justice in Spain, in which he accused the governor of being arbitrary and of having allowed himself to be influenced by the disturbing intrigues of Ignacio Canibell, an accountant in the Auditor's Office and a member of the board.

It is curious and illuminating to point out how Canibell aggravated the discord even more. According to Salias, its origin was due to the fact that Canibell disputed the order of the seating of members of the Municipal Council, who were also members of the vaccination board. The argument over who should have preferential seating—a byzantine argument that was very common during the colonial period—was evident in communications between the Municipal Council and the board. The governor backed Canibell, however, and the matter ended by the council forbidding the mayor and the attorney general to attend meetings of the board.

As a consequence of such disputes and intrigues the activities of the board declined markedly, to such an extent that many of its members no longer attended meetings. These included the vicar, who represented the archbishop, the regent, the administrators, Colonel Manuel del Fierro, and even, as Salias pointed out, the political secretary, Bello, who had tried unsuccessfully to resign the secretaryship when he refused to endorse the decree condemning Salias. There was enormous interest in the matter, but the complete record does not reveal the final results. We do know that following the dissent the governor designated the Count of San Javier, Rivas, Montenegro, and the medical members of the Medical Court to each take turns of one month to witness the weekly vaccination at the home of Aranda. As has been shown, however, the practical results could not have been more disheartening: the decline in the activities of the board was so great that the life of this interesting and useful body was gradually completely extinguished.

This incident happened only two years before the beginning of the revolution, which was already developing, whose cause Salias embraced with the most fervent patriotic ardor—he immortalized himself by writing the words to our national anthem *Gloria al Bravo Pueblo* (Glory to the Brave People). The question comes to mind: Is it not possible to attribute Salias's behavior to his anti-Spanish feelings? This incident, unpublished until now, and therefore unknown to Venezuelan historians, is worthy of study in the light of the new documents.

Perhaps the last thing that happened of medical interest was that, at the session of 27 February 1808, José Angel de Alamo informed the board of the circumstances under which smallpox had reappeared, and made proposals aimed at finding the hidden source of the contagion in order to prevent it from spreading and to allay the doubts that might discredit the vaccine. He also brought up the subject of whether the vaccination could have influenced the mildness of the smallpox cases recently discovered. According to Ildemaro Lovera, "Alamo raised an issue that many years later was to form a part of the modern concept of vaccination, i.e., the mildness of the symptoms of a disease in persons previously vaccinated, which at that time was only a supposition under study by the very people who had discovered virus vaccine."[42]

The final minutes in the book of records of the Central Vaccination Board are dated 9 April 1808. We do not actually know if the board's activities were continued by the successor to Governor de las Casas, Vicente de Emparán, who was in charge of the government of the province from 19 May 1809 until 19 April 1810. If they were not, then the board had an existence of four years, divided into two periods, as has been described.

It must be stated that Aranda, as director of vaccination, continued this work after the board was discontinued. But in our opinion, in spite of the internal problems that apparently led to its decline in the second period, basically the political ferment of 1810 probably had more influence than is thought in bringing about the board's lamentable end. In any case, it was the ten-year War of Independence that created the real barrier to the Vaccination Board continuing its work.

On 5 May 1810 the governor informed the secretary of the Supreme Council and the Office of Grace and Justice that he had ordered that every two weeks lists of infants baptized in that period should be sent to the vaccination office, as had been the custom in previous years. It was intended to continue the work carried out by the original board, but the long and bloody war completely upset the routine that was beginning to take shape.

Be that as it may, after dismissing Emparán, the Supreme Council that assumed the reins of government in Caracas decreed on 13 September 1810 that the Police Court should take full responsibility for the conservation, propagation, and perpetuation of the vaccine fluid, with the help of Aranda, who was confirmed as director of vaccination, with the right to vote at meetings.[43]

The history of the antismallpox vaccination campaign during its most important period, under the Republic, is material for another monograph. In 1815 the governor and captain-general, Salvador Moxó, reinstated the Central Board for a short period, and decreed that boards for vaccination be established in the principal provinces, with divisions in the capital cities.

It is of interest that Diaz was named secretary (scientific) and Arvelo secretary (administration) in this new organization.

EPILOGUE

The success of the introduction of the Jennerian vaccine to Venezuela, as indicated by the activities of the Central Vaccination Board, may be explained by a combination of the following factors:
- The innate receptivity of the inhabitants.
- Prior and thorough preparation of public opinion using techniques familiar to present-day teachers of health education.
- Unanimous and complete backing by the highest authorities led by the governor and captain-general, as well as the strong support of the ecclesiastical authorities, especially the priests.
- The cooperation of the local doctors, in particularly the outstanding performances of Jośe Domingo Díaz and Jośe Justo Aranda.
- A program based on the conservation and propagation of the fluid, in which the epidemiological measures taken were perfectly justified by present-day standards.
- The use of properly trained vaccinators.
- Strict avoidance of the old system of arm-to-arm vaccination.
- Venezuela's horrifying, almost Dantesque, history of smallpox, which, by the terrible toll it had taken over more than two centuries had made the population fearful, and, as a consequence, avid for any preventive method—it had previously accepted arm-to-arm vaccination without reservation.

If the invasions of General Francisco de Miranda presaged the change in the political structure of Venezuela, then, from the medical point of view, the creation and activities of the City Medical Office in Caracas, the famous expedition of Balmis, and the establishment of the Central Vaccination Board, were, during the period of transition from a colony to a Republic, the most important events that marked the culmination of the recently born sanitary science.

CONCLUSIONS

As an accomplishment without precedent, the Central Vaccination Board of Caracas (1804-08) was established in Spanish America as an immediate and direct consequence of the Balmis expedition. Its administration, a model in the field, served Balmis as an archetype and guide for the installation of similar bodies.[44]

Although the existence of the board had been mentioned by Venezuelan historians, the details of its operation, the magnitude of its activities, and the results of the vaccinations it carried out were not generally known. In capsulating this historical period, thanks to the board's minutes, its extraordinary significance in Venezuela has been brought to light, taking into consideration the period during which it was active and the resources at its command.

The achievements of the Central Vaccination Board and Venezuela's contribution to the history of the heroic expedition are so obvious that their positive value cannot be denied.

NOTES

1. Justino Fernandez, "La Expedición Científica de Alejandro Malaspina," in *Memorias del Primer Coloquio Mexicano de Historia de la Ciencia* (n.p.: n.p.): 101.

2. It is pleasing to find that the majority of writers are Latin American medical historians, including, among others: Eduardo García del Real, Anastacio Chinchilla, Hernández Morejón, P. D. Rodríquez Rivero, Rafael Dominguez, Aníbal Ruiz Moreno, Gonzalo Díaz de Yraola, Juan B. Lastres, Hipólito Unanue, Francisco Fernández del Castillo, Eliseo Cantón, Pedro Mallo, José Luis Molinari, Gualberto Arcos, Rafael Schiaffino, Vicuña Mackena, Mauro Madero, Andrés Soriano Lleras, Carlos Martínez Durán, Andrés Bello, Héctor García Chuecos, Ceferino Alegría y Alfonso Díaz Trigo.

3. Gonzalo Díaz de Yraola, *La Vuelta al Mundo de la Expedición de la Vacuna* (Seville: n.p. 1948).

4. Curious prevision induced by Dr. José Flores, author of the first plan, in chronological order, for the vaccination expedition: ". . . and in those places where there should be no Spanish or 'Latin' doctor available, it will be necessary to have the priests and missionaries do the vaccinations with the same ceremony that is used in baptism . . . and they should write the results in a book to be called *Vaccination* . . . "

5. Aníbal Ruiz Moreno, *Introducción de la Vacuna en América (Expedición de Balmis)* (Buenos Aires: n.p. 1947): Ch. II and III.

6. Royal order establishing the conservation and propagation of the vaccine. Document reproduced in Francisco Fernández del Castillo, p. 213.

7. General Archives of the Indies (Seville: General File 1558, folios 24 and 25).

8. Reproduction of the complete text of the Documentary Appendix (see pp. 178-81). It is almost identical to the project presented by Balmis to the viceroy of New Spain in Mexico City.

9. According to the testimony of Balmis at the time, it was believed that the vaccine not only protected against smallpox but had a favorable influence in the cure of certain skin diseases and many others, such as scrofula, rickets, leprosy, erysipelas, and even had preventive virtues against yellow fever and the bubonic plague. In an unpublished communication of José Domingo Díaz (General Archives of the Indies [Seville: General File 1558, no. 2, dated at Caracas, 21 March 1808]), he enumerated the great number and variety of diseases which at that time were considered to be affected by the vaccine. Therefore, at the meeting 9 November 1805, the governor and captain-general made a proposal, which was accepted, that Carlos del Pozo carry out experiments with the vaccine on local lepers and others in the Hospital for

Lepers in Caracas, "for which he should use the fluid from cows, as it is the strongest." At the session of 28 October 1805, a report had been submitted by the priest of Arenales testifying to the beneficial influence of the fluid, as observed in his parish, on various diseases such as the mumps, some venereal diseases, and ulcers.

10. Ruiz Moreno, *Introducción de la Vacuna* (See note 5).

11. Ricardo Archila, *La Expedición de Balmis en Venezuela* (Caracas: n.p., 1969): 17.

12. *Expedición de la Vacuna*, Minutes of 2 June 1804, Archives of the Illustrious Municipal Council of the Federal District, Caracas.

13. The magnificent mansion of the Count of San Javier was built in 1736 in the heart of Caracas, on the spot where today is situated the Ministry of Education. In addition to the meetings of the Vaccination Board, sessions were held there of the Supreme Board of Caracas, keeper of the rights of Ferdinand VII (1910); in 1811 the deputies to the First Congress of Venezuela met in its halls. Before its demolition it was occupied successively by the *Imprenta Nacional, El Eco Venezolano, and El Nuevo Diario.*

14. On 22 June 1804 King Charles IV extended his approval of the activities of the Central Vaccination Board of Caracas.

15. Archila, *Expedición de Balmis* (See note 11).

16. At the beginning of 1808 the commander of Barinas asked for scabs from smallpox sores in order to vaccinate the population of his province. The central board refused, ordering him to apply to Guanare or another city where it might be more convenient to obtain fresh fluid.

17. The systematic training of local doctors in all details of vaccination was considered a fundamental necessity. During his stay in Caracas, Balmis dedicated himself to the subject: "Balmis has not wasted any necessary time or effort to give the professors of this city and elsewhere who have come to him the information they may not have known, indicating to them clearly the principles of vaccination. These instructions were necessary because, once he left, the king's objectives might have been thwarted had the fluid been left in the hands of ignorant or absentminded professors. For that reason, I have taken particular pains to stimulate them and to induce them to learn in detail, so that hereafter they may observe and contribute to others, observing the warnings and precautions established for the purpose." Excerpted from the report of the captain-general of Caracas on the arrival of the Royal Expedition. General Archives of the Indies (Seville: General File 1558, no. 2)

18. Díaz, *Vuelta de la Expedición* (See note 3).

19. During the session of 19 October 1805 the application of Francisco Rico, vaccinator for the district of Macuto for a salary to be assigned him, was read. It was agreed that the lieutenant of Macuto should take up a collection from the affluent inhabitants and landowners who voluntarily wished to contribute. When vaccinations were started in Maracaibo, "a doctor with a salary of 15 pesos monthly was placed in charge of the conservation, and the salary was charged to funds of the inhabitants of the city." General Archives of the Indies (Seville: General File 1559).

20. By order of Governor Guevara y Vasconcelos, between late 1802 and early 1803 Díaz carried out vaccinations, with negative results, based on fluid taken from cows in the district of Victoria.

21 Alexander Freiherr von Humboldt, *Voyage aux régions équinoxiales du nouveau continent* (n.p.: 1805).

22. Because it is of singular interest, we reproduce here Díaz's statement of 22 December 1804 concerning Pozo's discovery: "On 15 November, Mr. Carlos del Pozo informed me of his series of experiments. At the beginning of 1804 he obtained the first printed news in these provinces which explained the nature, qualities, effects and manner of using the vaccine fluid. Just as he had made arrangements to take it from the udders of cows, there came news of the arrival of the director, Francisco Xavier Balmis. Abandoning a project that now seemed superfluous, and being particularly interested to learn about the character and circumstances of the admirable pustules, he sent a man to Caracas. After being vaccinated, the man returned promptly to his own town and Pozo carried out several vaccinations with the fluid taken from

his arm with great success. Later came the president's order forbidding this operation because of the false vaccinations that were beginning to appear, which were being carried out by ignorant people full of a regrettable enthusiasm. Pozo suspended the vaccinations he had been performing periodically and returned to his original ideas and tried to obtain information that would enable him to act with assurance. His advisors induced him to continue his investigations, however, and one of his friends presented him with a cow with characteristic sores. He took fluid from the sores and applied it to the arms of two children he had secretly prepared beforehand. On the fourth day after the application, there started to appear in each incision a slight button, depressed in its center, that grew, and pain was felt in the armpits. On the tenth and eleventh days there was some delirium, nausea, and symptoms of lesser consideration; during this time the pustules had the same appearance as those produced by the fluid brought by the Royal Expedition. On the thirteenth and fourteenth days all the symptoms disappeared and the vaccinated parties recovered completely. With the fluid taken on the prescribed day Pozo vaccinated eight other people, and they acquired pustules that were the same as those of the Royal Expedition, without the terrible symptoms that the first group showed. At this time there arrived in town a vaccinator sent by your excellency, and for this reason Pozo ceased his useful investigations and extended to your excellency his deep thanks for having selected him. When the months of June and July came around, which was when this affliction became generalized in the cows, Pozo would continue his experimentations, rectify his observations, remit the fluid, and, when it became necessary, sacrifice his rest to carry out this work in order to be worthy of the confidence you have been kind enough to bestow on him." General Archives of the Indies (Seville: General File 1558).

23. Archila, *Expedición de Balmis* (See note 11).

24. *El Médico José Domingo Díaz Contemplado por Otro Médico en el Año Setenta del Siglo XX* (Caracas: n.p., 1970).

25. In the university archives we have found twenty tables signed by Dr. José Domingo Díaz: there are eight separate ones from May to December 1804, which are partial; and one general one dated 22 January 1805, titled "Demonstration of those Vaccinated in this Province from May to December 1804 According to the Lists So Far Received." It contains the enumeration of 31 cities and towns, with squares indicating kinds: white, brown, Indian, Negro; and ages: from birth to one month, to legal age, to 100 years. The total amount is 12,450....Ten tables, from February to December 1805 containing 7,285 vaccinated, carry these notes: "1) Since the departure of the Royal Expedition until yesterday there have been vaccinated, according to the lists, 56,552 persons; 2) vaccination has been carried out in 74 places, including the capital. (Caracas, December 13th, 1805, José Domingo Díaz).... Every partial table contains the indication of its squares and the subtotals with observations.... As an unusual observation, we may take notice that one of the partial tables (that of 13 July 1805,) carries this note: '1) Mr. Miguel Barrios, from el Baúl, 100 years of age, had an excellent vaccination without the slightest trouble." In Rafael Domínguez, "La Vacuna en Venezuela," *Gazeta Médica de Caracas* XXXVI, no. 2 (1929): 19-25.

26. In a report presented by Díaz to the Central Vaccination Board on 15 March 1808, he stated: "In the four years that have elapsed since the departure of the Royal Expedition... there have been vaccinations in 107 cities, towns, and villages to 104,619 people." The population of Venezuela in the year 1807 was 975,972.

27. The following is a bibliographic index on smallpox and vaccination for the period 1802-10: *From José Domingo Díaz*: 1) Opinion of the project for the extinction of smallpox presented by the royal physician Tamariz to the governor and captain-general Vasconcelos, 19 May 1802. (Reproduced in *Catalog of the Donación Villanueva*, National Academy of Medicine, vol. 1, p. 209). 2) Report on the procedure for the propagation of the vaccine (in collaboraton with Santiago Limardo and Ignacio Canibell) 12 May 1804. 3) Instructions for recognizing the vaccine and for carrying out the vaccination, by Díaz and Vicente Salias, 29 May 1804. (Taken from the instructions sent from Spain and adapted to our circumstancces and our climate by these authors.) 4) Report on the state and progress of vaccination in the country, the number of vaccinations, and the useful discoveries of Carlos del Pozo (presented before the

Central Vaccination Board on 19 October 1805). 5) Special report to the board of 6 October 1804 to inform the king about the difficulties, obstacles, problems, etc. relative to vaccination. 6) Report on the ways smallpox infection is preserved in the graves of smallpox victims (in collaboration with Salias), 23 February 1805, (in regard to the report by José Antonio Montenegro.) 7) Estimate of the number of people who would probably have died of smallpox if they had not received the benefit of the vaccine, 14 December 1805. (Read before the Central Vaccination Board on 1 February 1806.) 8) Report on the activities of the vaccination board from October 1805 to March 1808, on the state, decadence or progress, of the conservation of the vaccine fluid in the capital and in the provinces, and on the phenomena that during said period of time have been observed or that confirm previous observations, 21 March 1808.

28. Bibliographic index on smallpox and vaccination for the period 1802-10. *From Vicente Salias*: 1) Report on the manner of perpetuating in the capital and the provinces the vaccination fluid in such a manner as to assure its legitimacy and permanence (in collaboration with Montenegro and Xavier Ustábriz, 12 May 1804.) 2) Reflections on the propagation of the vaccination fluid; report he produced as an appendix to that read at the 12 May session, on the manner of preserving the vaccine germ (presented to the vaccination board on 19 May.) Observations I have carried out on the vaccine, 24 April 1804. (This refers to the commission given him by Balmis to examine the first sixty-four persons vaccinated on Holy Friday of that year.) 3) See work in collaboration with *Díaz*. 4) Reflections on the false vaccine, 20 February 1808. *From Felipe Tamariz*: 1) Observations I have carried at the Royal Hospital of San Lazaro of the City of Santiago de León de Caracas, with the leprous patients that were vaccinated on 7 April 1804. (Reproduced in Rodríguez Rivero, *Historia Médica de Venezuela* (n.p.: n.d.): 76 ff. 2) Report on the way to eliminate the contagion of natural smallpox in the capital and other parts of the province (in collaboration with José Ignacio Moreno and José Joaquín Hernández), 19 May 1804. *From Santiago Limardo*: Report on ways to preserve the vaccine fluid without having to depend on ordinary arm-to-arm vaccination, (in collaboraton with José Antonio Montenegro), 9 June 1804. *From Montenegro*: Report on the danger represented by the opening of the graves that contained corpses of smallpox victims, 1 December 1804. *From Lawyer Manuel Benard*: Report on the persons inoculated by me, 26 April 1804. (This refers to the vaccination, not the inoculation, of smallpox). *From Diego Luis Pereyra*, a surgeon in Valencia: Copy of the diary I keep of the vaccinations that I perform in this city, together with observations on the effects of the fluids on the course of the disease, 4 May 1804. *From José Justo Aranda*: Conservation of the vaccine fluid, May 1804. *From José Angel Alamo*: Reflections on a case of smallpox, February 1808. *From José Joaquín Hernández*: On means to prevent the false vaccine, 1808. *From Antonio Gomez*: On ways to prevent the false vaccine, March 1808. *From Francisco Javier Ustáriz*: 1) Report on the probability of finding the cowpox in the province of Caracas, 5 January 1805. 2) Report on the necessity of abolishing the practice of burials in churches, 5 January 1805.

29. Decree of Governor Juan de las Casas read at the inaugural session: "Junta Central de la Vacuna, 1804-08," session of 16 November 1807.

30. Andrés Bello was at that time second clerk of the Secretariat of the Captaincy-General.

31. General Archives of the Indies (Seville: General File 1558).

32. The Book of Minutes of the Central Vaccination Board contains frequent complaints from vaccinators, some requesting salaries, others requesting raises.

33. Toward the end of February or beginning of March 1808, news was received of the formation of the Subaltern Board of Vaccination of Puerto Cabello, which was approved.

34. Ricardo Archila, *História de la Sanidad en Venezuela*, vol. I (Caracas: n.p., 1956).

35. *Obras Completas de Andrés Bello*, vol. XX (Caracas: Ministerio de Educación, Comisión Editora de las Obras Completas de Andrés Bello, 1957): Appendix.

36. The autographical reproduction is admirable. According to the inscription, it was "made by special process for the reproduction of autographs and old manuscripts" in the print and lithography shop of Felix Rasco.

37. Archila, *Sanidad en Venezuela* (See note 34): 62.

38. Andrés Bello, *Oda a la Vacuna*. In Archila, *Expedición de Balmis* (See note 15): 23.
39. Communication from Díaz to the Central Vaccination Board, 21 March 1808. General Archives of the Indies (Seville: General File 1558).
40. Aranda later petitioned for a certification of his good services, which the board awarded.
41. The documentation consulted for this information is in the General Archives of the Indies (Seville: General File 1558). It entails the following documents: "Reflections on the False Vaccine" by Vicente Salias; communication from Salias to the minister of grace and justice, 29 March 1808; communication from Díaz to the vaccination board, 21 March 1808; and representation of the captain-general of Venezuela to the minister of grace and justice, 26 March 1808.
42. Ildemaro Lovera, *História de una Oligarquía* (Caracas: n.p., 1965): 138.
43. In 1812, the year of his death, Aranda was still acting as examiner of romance languages and keeper of the vaccine fluid.
44. R. Gickhorn and H. Schadewaldt, "Sobre la Introducción de la Vacuna Antivariolosa en América," in *Ensayos Históricas*, Homage to Tomás Romay (Havana: n.p., 1968): 407.

DOCUMENTARY APPENDIX

On the Establishment of a Central Vaccination Board in Caracas*

The following is the edited document in which Francisco Xavier Balmis proposed the establishment of a Central Vaccination Board in Caracas on 15 April 1804.

1. Experience has often shown that the vaccine humor ... is extinguished more or less promptly. If it is desired to keep and perpetuate it in a province, it is imperative that a board be established. It should be subordinate to and under the immediate authority of the government, and be composed of four to six persons respected in the neighborhood who have shown a concern about public welfare; and an equal number, more or less, of professors of medicine and surgery to observe and enforce the observation of a fixed and inalterable regimen that will be capable of filling such a salutary purpose. It is my belief that the captain-general and the illustrious bishop of this diocese should ... constitute themselves protectors of this beneficent congregation, and that the mayor of first election and the attorney-general, among other voters now in office and those who may come in the future ... should be members of a body that promotes and represents the rights and benefits of these inhabitants.

2. This board will have a vice-president designated by the captain-general, and two secretariats, of which one will have the obligation to take care of the correpsondence that may come up with the other provinces and towns in the interior ... with respect to government, economic affairs, means of supplying the fluid, and other nonscientific matters. The other should be a doctor who should [record] everything pertaining to the practice of vaccination and its effects, the observations made about all of which he is to inform the board ... so that they may discuss and agree on the correct procedure.

3. The Central Vaccination Board will hold its meetings one day a week, when

---

* Copied from *Libro en que se Asientan los Asientan los Acuerdos de la Junta Central de la Vacuna* (Caracas: Archives of the Illustrious Municipal Council of the Federal District).

they will discuss not only the examination, inspection, and condition of those vaccinated during the previous week, but various events in the other towns and provinces . . . of which this capital is head: the need to send vaccine to other places, or to have their doctors or interested parties come here to be instructed in the practice of vaccination and the knowledge required to use it with dexterity.

4. A place will be selected . . . in which to hold the meetings and to give weekly the public arm-to-arm vaccinations, with the object of keeping the fluid . . . free of any adulteration or degeneration, so that it may be perpetuated and natural smallpox completely eradicated. To attain this [objective] it will be necessary to adapt the means that the government, of itself or on petition of the board, may consider fit and capable of extending to the entire dominion, either by sending professors to those places where there are none or by bringing them from those towns to carry and propagate the vaccine, so that the present generation and the newborn may be free of the danger of smallpox . . . .

5. Two professors on . . . the board should practice the public vaccination without charge to the people who receive this benefit, until, on collecting some funds, they may be recompensed for their work as seems just: all shall take turns, by months, not only to distribute the work but to acquire the agility . . . that the repeated and observed operation that is entrusted to them will afford.

6. No member of the board will receive any payment except for the gratification of . . . this honorable, praiseworthy occupation recommended by the king, which cedes its benefits to humanity and public health, to which all of us should of good grace make some sacrifice.

7. The merely inquisitive will not be permitted to vaccinate, nor will any other person who has not obtained previous written permission from the board, which will be charged with ensuring that false vaccinations do not occur, because these do not in any way protect from smallpox, and are easily spread due to the ignorance of the vaccinator. . . .

8. Considering that the king's orders direct the joining of the spiritual and temporal powers for the success of his pious ideas, the secretary of the board will each month present to the captain-general a statement of the number of those vaccinated and other events occurring during that time, and will appeal to his high protection so that he will issue the orders deemed necessary for the preservation of the precious treasure that by his majesty's order is now placed in his hands, and that . . . the same be done with the very reverend bishop, so that he may order all the venerable priests in his entire diocese to send news and make inscriptions in the parochial books on children that are born.

9. Whenever there should be news that, in spite of these precautions and others the magistrates may take, smallpox has broken out in . . . the province, the board, in accord with its president, will name an intelligent vaccinator to take the precious fluid . . . and, through its use, break the smallpox contagion, paying him out of the public funds of the town being benefited . . . it shall be warmly recommended that he instruct the local doctor or [other] person . . . in everything concerning the practice of vaccination.

10. One of the principal duties of the board is to have correspondents in all parts of this captaincy-general to observe whether the herds of cows have any vaccine sores in the teats of their udders, or cowpox, as it is called in England . . . particularly during spring and autumn. These correspondents . . . should be doctors who are capable of making vaccination trials with the pus from the cowpox, and who can decide whether the results are the true vaccine that . . . has been brought to you by this Royal Expedition. But if there is a lack of professors, [the correspondents] may be the most learned inhabitants of known zeal and love for the welfare of their fellow men. . . .

11. Having established through constant experimentation that the precious vaccine not only enjoys the virtue of protecting against smallpox but has cured many skin diseases, that it also improves and strengthens the weak constitution of the vaccinated, and lastly, that it opposes the development of scrofula and rickets . . . the board should experiment with [those afflicted with] elephantiasis and St. Anthony's fire, [diseases] that are so abundant in this continent. The latest observations made in Constantinople have proved that this admirable fluid is also a protection against the plague, and it is to be expected that it may also protect against the black vomit and yellow fever, putrid, malignant and pestilential diseases that only differ from the true Turkish plague in the greater degree of their malignity; . . . it may be that a specific could be obtained against these cruel diseases that cause such ravages, particularly among those shortly arrived from Europe.

12. The professor in charge of the secretariat will enter in his book the new discoveries that may be made and take care to communicate them to the director of the Royal Vaccination Expedition, so he may enter them into the log of his voyage, which he is to publish by order of His Majesty, and in which will be mentioned the name and circumstance of the author and the comments he may make, so that he may be distinguished and appreciated according to his merit . . . and that to him may befall the compensation that His Majesty may consider just, according to his offer.

Francisco Xavier Balmis

Caracas, 15 April 1804

* * * *

Testimony of José Domingo Díaz and Santiago Limardo, professors of medicine entrusted by the Central Vaccination Board with the examination of individuals who are to perform vaccinations in the province of Caracas.

We have examined, according to the intentions of the Board, Senor José Escalona, for the jurisdiction of Barinas and other areas that he applies for,* and, having performed, in theory and practice, before us all that which we believe necessary to show his ability: We judge him to have the capacity to

---

* On 26 June the president extended Senor Escalona's license allowing him to vaccinate not only in the city of Barinas, but in Guanare and the towns of Ospino and Araure.

proceed with judgment and safety in the operation of which he intends to take charge.

José Domingo Díaz
Santiago Limardo

Caracas, 22 June 1804

* * * *

Testimony of Vicente Salias and José Justo de Aranda.

We certify to the best of our ability, before the persons and Tribunals that may see this document, and in virtue of the decree of his Lordship, the President, Governor and Captain-general, and local gentlemen of the Central Vaccination Board, that we have examined Senor Manuel Pantoja in theory and practice and found him capable of carrying out vaccinations, as well as being able to distinguish the bad pustules from the good ones. As evidence we present this document, signed in Caracas on 9 February 1808.

Vicente Salias
José Justo de Aranda

Caracas, 9 February 1808

PARTICIPANTS

Ricardo Archila, M.D., M.P.H.
Urbanizacion las Palmas
Caracas, Venezuela

Gustavo Beyhaut Ph.D.
Instituto de Economia y Planificacion
Universidad de Chile
Santiago, Chile

Charles R. Boxer Ph.D.
The Lilly Library
Indiana University
Bloomington, Indiana

Fernando Cabieses, M.D.
Director
Peruvian Museum
   of Health Sciences
Lima, Peru

Donald B. Cooper, Ph.D.
Department of History
Ohio State University
Columbia, Ohio

Francisco Guerra M.D.
Madrid, Spain

E. Croft Long, M.B., B.S., Ph.D.
Project Hope
Guatemala City, Guatemala

Joaquin V. Luco, M.D.
Professor of Neurophysiology
Facultad de Medicina y Ciencias Biologico
Universidad Catolica de Chile
Santiago, Chile

Jaime Mendiola Gomez, M.D.
Head
Department of Microbiology
Universidad Autonoma de Guadalajara
Guadalajara, Mexico

John Horace Parry, Ph.D.
Gardiner Professor of Oceanic History and Affairs
Harvard University
Cambridge, Massachusetts

Vilma Piedrahita, M.D.
Facultad de Medicina
Universidad de Antioquia
Medellin, Colombia

Lycurgo de C. Santos Filho, M.D.
Campinas, Sao Paulo, Brazil

John B. deC. M. Saunders, M.D., M.D.
Emeritus Professor
Department of the History of Health Sciences
University of California
San Francisco, California

Virgil C. Scott, M.D.*
The Rockefeller Foundation
New York, New York

Andres Soriano Lleras, M.D.
Associate Professor of Microbiology
Facultad de Medicina
Universidad Nacional de Colombia
Bogota, Colombia

---

* Retired

PARTICIPANTS

Carlos Tejada, M.D.
Director
Instituto de Nutricion de Centro America y Panama
Guatemala City, Guatemala

Gabriel Velazquez Palau, M.D.
The Rockefeller Foundation
Cali, Colombia

Robert B. Watson, M.D.
Emeritus Professor of Parasitology
School of Public Health
University of North Carolina
Chapel Hill, North Carolina

INDEX

Academia Brasílica dos Renascidos, 106
Academia de los Felices, 106
De Accidentibus (Avecina), 89
Ackernecht, E.H., 3
Acosta, José de, on potato as Mayan food, 69
administration of medical practice, Brazil, 103-04
De Agritudinibus (Avecina), 89
aid, mutual, in ancient Peru, 43-44
Alamo, José Antonio, 163
Amor, Rosendo, 95
anatomy, pre-Columbian knowledge of, 7
Anchieta, José de, 100, 109
Andrade, Rodrigo Enríquez de, 125
anesthesia, pre-Columbian, 9
Angelica University, 117
animals
  in Mayan diet, 61-68, 79, 80
  in Mayan symbolism, 66
Anthropological Society of Berlin, 24, 25-26
Anthropology, pre-Columbian, 5
Antonio Gómez, José, 161, 163
Aphorisms (Hippocrates), 89
Aranda, José Justo, 147, 151, 159, 163
Araucanians, medical profession, 6
archaeology, American, 1-3
Archila, Ricardo, 127
Arctic hysteria, 9
Argentina, colonial medical education, 125
Arias, Domingo, 90
armadillo, as Mayan food, 63, 65
Aróstegui y Escoto, José Joaquin de, 118
De Arte Curativa ad Glaucomen (Galileo), 89
arthritis, in ancient Peru, 18-19

Ashmead, A., 24, 25, 27
Arvelo, Carlos, 168
Ataide, António de, 135
Atriesta, José de, 116
autochthonous diseases, pre-Columbian, 9
avocado, as Mayan food, 71
Aztecs, 2
  epidemics, 10
  knowledge of anatomy, 7
  medical profession, 6-7
  obstetrics, 9
  pathology and diagnosis, 7-8
  teaching of medicine, 88

Badian Codex, 88
Badiano, Juan, 88
Balmis expedition, 127, 142-43
  activities interrupted, 162
  bibliographic balance, 161-62
  board created, 143-47, 178-81
  board reorganized, 162-64
  board supporters, 158-59
  board terminated, 168-72
  cowpox discovery given priority, 156-58
  general measures, 155-56
  initial activities, 147-49
  numerical balance, 161
  persuasive and coerive measures, 149-50
  vaccination fluid conservation, 150-52
  vaccine distribution, 152-55
  work program, 164-65
The Balmis Expedition in Venezuela (Archila), 150
Barrios, Juan de, 91
Bartolache, José Ignacio, 93
bartonellosis, 9

Baz, Gustavo 96
beans
  growing and consuming, 61
  varieties, 60
beekeepers, Mayan, and festivals, 73
bees, varieties, 72-73
Bellow, Andrés, 125, 162, 163, 165-66
Beltran de Santa Rose, P., 7
Benítez, José Ma., 94
Berson, Robert, 129
Betanzos, Juan Sotelo de, 90
Bettencourt, Anibal Cymbron Barbosa, 132
birds, as Mayan food, 63-64, 65-66
Blaya, Attorney General, 120
Bohorquez, José, 117
Bolivar, Simon, 159
bone disorders, ancient Peru, 18-19
Bravo, Francisco, 90
Brazil
  administration of medical practice, 103-04
  clinical school, 107
  Dutch medicine, 104-05
  first medical professionals, 98-99
  Holy Houses of Mercy, 101
  Jesuit healers, 99-100, 110-11
  land and diseases, 97-98
  medical organizations, 106-07
  medical professionals, 101-03
  mixture of races, 99
  sanitary measures, 104
  scientific literature, 105-06
  scientific research, 104
Brief Treatise on Medicine (Farfán), 90
Brief Treatise on Surgery, and Knowledge and Cause of Certain Diseases (Farfán), 90
"browse" (ramón) tree, 71
Buenaventura, Jacinto, 117

Caballero, Don José Antonio, 145
Caballero y Góngora, Viceroy, 117
Cabral, Pedro Alvares, 97

Cagiao, Joaquín, 123
Cagigal, Governor, 153
Caldas, Francisco José de, 126
Cameron, J.W., 56
Campins y Ballester, Lorenzo, 125
cancer, in ancient Peru, 20-21
Cancino, Vicente Román, 115, 116
Canibell, Ignacio, 147, 148,163
cannibalism, 7, 62
Caraza, Rafaél, 95
carbohydrates, in pre-Columbian diet, 4
Cárdenas, Lucas de, 90
Carmona y Valle, Manuel, 95
Carpio, Manuel, 94
Carrasquilla, 25
Carter, H. R., 4
Castilla, Pedro Fernández de, 115
Castro Santos, José Manuel de, 102, 103
catharsis, pre-Columbian, 12-13
De Causis (Avecina), 89
Caycedo y Flórez, Fernando, 118, 119, 120
Center for Population Research, 131
Cesar, Luís, 132
Charles II, 125
Charles III, 126
Charles IV, 118, 125
Charles V, 88, 124
Chávez, Ignacio, 96
chewing gum, 70
children, Mayan, care and feeding, 77-79
Chile, colonial medical education, 125
Chile, University of, 125
chocolate and cocoa, 73-74
Cieza, P., 36
Cisneros, Diego, 91
Clavijo y Clavijo, Salvador, 136
clinical school, Brazil, 107
Cobo, P. Bernabé, 35, 48, 51
  on cannibalism, 62
cocoa

growing of, 73-74
as monetary unit, 75
Codex Badianus, 8, 12
Codex Dresdensis, 55, 66
Codex Peresianus, 57-58
Codex Tro-Cortesianus, 67, 73
De cognocendis et curandis morbis (Boerhaave), 123
Columbia, medical education in, 112-23, 125, 129-31
corn
  consumption, 59-60
  divine manifestation, 55-56
  growing system, 57-58
  origin of, 56-57
cornbread, 60
Cortés, Juan José, 116
Courtois, Juan José, 115
cowpox, Balmis expedition priority given to discovery of, 156-58
Crespo, Diego, 117
Cueto, Damián Gonzáles, 90
cultural trends, pre-Columbian, 4-6
Cursus Medicus Mexicanus (Salgado), 93

Dabbert, O., 18, 36
daily life and habitual food, Maya, 75-77
dancing mania, 9
deer, as Mayan food, 65, 68
de la Calancha, Antonio, 22
de la Cruz, José, 114
de la Cruz, Martín, 88
  on diagnosis, 8
de la Fuente, Juan, 89
de las Casas, Juan, 148, 159, 163, 164, 169
Del Valle University (Cali), 129-31
dental problems, ancient Peru, 36
diagnosis
  in ancient Peru, 51-52
  and pathology, pre-Columbian, 7-8
Diálogo entre un Vizcaíno y un Montenés, 136

Dias Pimenta, Miguel, 106
Diaz, Francisco, 112
Diaz, José Domingo, and Balmis expedition, 147-68
Diaz del Castillo, Bernal, 67
  on Mayan meats, 68
Diaz Quijano, José Gregorio, 118
diet
  and nutrition, Mayan, 79-81, 85-87
  pre-Columbian, 3-4
diseases
  attitudes in ancient Peru toward, 44-47
  colonial Brazil, 97-98
  nutritional, and diet, 80-81
  pre-Columbian, 3, 4, 9-12
  transmission, ancient Peru, 47-50
dogs, as Mayan food, 62-63
Don Manuel I, 97
drink, alcoholic, in pre-Columbian civilizations, 4
Drugs, pre-Columbian, 3, 12
Dutch, in Brazil, 104-05
Dutch West India Company, 105

Eaton, G.F., 23
Echezuría, Alejandro, 163
Ecuador, colonial medical education in, 124
endocrinological disorders, ancient Peru, 27
Enriques de Andrade, Licenciado Rodrigo, 112-14
epidemic diseases, pre-Columbian, 4, 10-12
Epidemics (Hippocrates), 89
Erario Mineral (Ferreira), 138-40
Escobedo, Pedro, 94
Esens, Guilherme Escoph de, 132-38
Eslaba y Caballero, Rafaél de, 114
Espinosa de los Monteros, José Félix, 153, 165
Esteinffer, Juan de, 93
Estete, Miguel de, 32

Expedición de la Vacuna, 143
eye disorders, in ancient Peru, 35-36

famine, Maya, 81-82
Faras, Juan, 97
Farfán, Augustín, 90
Farfán, García de, 90
Ferreira, Luís Gomes, 138-40
Ferreira da Rosa, João, 106, 111
festivals, Mayan, 67, 73, 79
fevers, in ancient Peru, 20-21
Fierro, Manuel, 147
Fierro, Pérez Cabeza de, 93
fish, in Mayan diet, 64, 66
Flora Cumanensis, 126
Flora Mexicana (Sessé and Mocino), 127
Flores, José Felipe, 150
Fracastorius, 16
Froes, Antonio, 117
fruits, in Mayan diet, 70-72
Fuentes, Francisco de, 114
Fuentes y Guzmán, F.A. de, on beans, 61

Gaceta de Caracas, 161
Gaceta de Madrid, 157-58
Gage, Tomas
 on chocolate, 73, 74
 on goiter in Maya, 80-81
 on preparation of deer meat, 68
 on preparation of tortillas, 59
Galileo Galilei, 89
García, José, 91
García, Miguel, 93
García Bedoya, H., 36
García Frías, J.E., 28
Garcilaso, Inca, 43, 46, 50, 51
General Anthology of All Diseases, (Esteinffer), 93
god-germ concept, ancient Peru, 50-51
goiter
 in Incas, 9
 in Maya, 80-81

Gonzalez Holquin, D., 7
Gorman, Miguel, 125
Goss, Charles, 129
Grases, Pedro, 165
Guairior, Viceroy, 118
guava, as Mayan food, 72
Guevara y Vasconcelos, Manuel de, 144, 158, 163
Gutierrez y Robledo, 93
Guzman, Gonzalez, 96

Hamperl, H., 33
Hawkins, Sir Richard, 135, 136
Hernández, Francisco, 12, 90, 105, 126, 127
Hernández, José Joaquín, 147, 148, 161
Herrejón, González, 96
Herrera, Antonio de, 22, 32
Hippocrates, 89
História da medicina no Brasil (Santos Filho), 108, 109
História de la Sanidad en Venezuela (Archila), 165
História Naturalis Brasiliae, 105, 106
De História Plantarum Nova Hispaniae (Hernandez), 90
hog (peccari), as Mayan food, 65
Holy Houses of Mercy, Brazil, 101
honey, as Mayan food, 72-73
Hooten, E., 23
Hospital de las Galeras de la Iglesia de San Juan de Letrán, 137
Hrdlicka, A., 18-19, 33
Huamán-Poma, F., 27, 36, 38, 46-47
human sacrifices, pre-Columbian, 5
Humphreys, G.H., 129
hunting, Mayan, 63, 64
hyperostosis, spongy, in ancient Peru, 33-34

Ibarra, Francisco de, 156, 158, 163
Ignacio, Manuel, 117
iguana, as Mayan food, 64

immolation, pre-Columbian, 5
Imperial College of Santa Cruz, 88
Incas
  epidemics, 10
  knowledge of anatomy, 7
  medical profession, 6
  mutual aid, 43-44
  pathology and diagnosis, 8
  psychotherapy, 13-14
  surgery, 9
Inciarte, Governor, 151
Institute of Medical Sciences (Mexico), 94
Instrucción de Generales y Almirantes de Flotas de la Carreira de Indias, 136
Instructions for the Curing of the Sick Afflicted with Smallpox Epidemics (Bartolache), 93
International Congress on Leprosy, 25
Isla, Miguel de, 115, 118, 119, 121
Isnardi, Francisco, 163
Izquierdo, José, 96
Izquierdo, Julián de, 165

Jesuits, in Brazil, 99-100, 101, 110
Jews, in Brazil, 104, 110-11
Jiménez de la Espada, 27
Jove, José García, 94

kaika, 39-41
Keevil, J.J., 136
Kellogg (W.K.) Foundation, 129
Kidder, A.V., 23

Landa, Diégo de, Bishop
  on cultivation of corn, 58, 59
  on food, 86
  on game animals as Mayan food, 63-64
  on honey bees, 72
  on Mayan festival, 67
  on Mayan women, 76
  on Yucatan trees, 71
Lapham, Max E., 129

Lasa, Lorenzo, 147
Lastres, J.B., 18
Latin America
  colonial medical educaton, 124-29
  community research, 130
  scientific expeditions, 126-27
leishmaniasis, cutaneous, 9
Leon, N., 9
leprosy, 16-17, 24-25, 27
Leuftink, A., 135
Liceaga, Casimiro, 94
Liceaga, Eduardo, 95
Lilly Library, Indiana University, 138-39
Limardo, Santiago, 147, 148, 161
Linnaeus, Carolus, 126
literature, scientific, Brazil, 105-06
Loayza, Fray Rodrigo, 23-24
Loefling, Peter, 126
López, Alonso, 90
López, Gregorio, 91
López, Juan, 112
López de Gomara, Francisco, 22, 36
López Méndez, Luis, 151, 152
López Ruíz, Sebastián, 118
Loza, Leopoldo Río de la, 95
Lucio, Rafáel, 95
lymphogranuloma, in ancient Peru, 22

Magaña, Diego de, 90
malaria, in ancient Peru, 20-21
Malaspina, Alejandro, 142
Malaspina expedition, 127
Maldonado, A., 39
malformations, congenital, in ancient Peru, 27-28
man, corn as creative element of, 55-56
manatee, as Mayan food, 64
Mangelsdorf, P.C., 56
Manrique, Antonio González, 116, 117
Marcgraf, George, 105
Marine Hospital, Cartagena, 115
Martínez de los Ríos, Diego, 90
Mas, Father, 114

Master Juan, 97
Masustegui, Miguel de, 116
Materia Medica (Boerhaave), 122
Maya, 1
  bee honey, 72-73
  child care and feeding, 77-79
  cocoa and chocolate, 73-75
  daily life and habitual food, 75-77
  diet and nutrition, 79-81
  epidemics, 10
  famine, 81-82
  food: of animal origin, 61-68
  food: beans, 60-61
  food: corn, 55-60
  food: fruits, 70-72
  food: vegetables, 69-70
  hunting, 66-68
  medical profession, 6
  pathology and diagnosis, 8
  salt, 75
McCurdy, G., 23
meal, principal Mayan, 76-77
meat, Mayan preparation and consumption of, 68
De Medica Artis Constitutione (Galileo), 89
medical education
  Aztecs, 88
  Latin America, 127-29
  preventive medicine and public health, 129-30
  See also Mexico, medical education
medical history, pre-Columbian, 3
medical organizations, Brazil, 106-07
medical profession, pre-Columbian, 6-7
medical professionals, Brazil, 101-03
Medicinal Anthology (Fierro), 93
Medicaments (Boerhaave), 122
medicine
  Dutch, in Brazil, 104-05
  teaching in colonial Colombia, 112-23

  See also pre-Columbian medicine; Peru
Melo, Gastón, 95
Mendieta, J. de, 7, 13, 89
Mendinueta, Viceroy, 119
Mendoza, Antonio de, 89, 124
mental functions, ancient Peru, 36-39
mental illness, ancient Peru, 39-43
El Murcurio Volante, 93
mercury, in ancient Peru, 32-33
Methodo Modendi (Boerhaave), 122
Mexican Revolution, 95
Mexican War of Independence, 93
Mexico, medical education
  beginnings, 88-91
  colonial, 124
  curricular changes, 94-96
  Office of Royal Physicians, 91-92
  protests and reforms, 93-94
  Royal College of Surgeons, 92-93
Mexico, University of, 90
Military Medical School, Mexico, 95
Miranda, Francisco de, 162
Mochicas, 2
Mocino, José María, 127
Molina, C. de, 43
Montaña, Luis, 93
Montanéz, Andrés, 93
Montenegro, José Antonio, 147
Montesinos, Francisco de, 35
Moodie, R., 18, 36
De Morbis Curandi (Galileo), 89
Moreau de la Sarthe Treaty, 143-44
Moreno, J.I., 147, 148, 163
Moreno, Juan de Torres, 91
Moreno, Manuel Antonio, 93
Moreno y Escandón, Francisco, 117, 118
Morley, S.G., 56
  on corn, 57, 82
  on Mayan evening meal, 76
Morúa, M. de, 48
Mosquera y Figueroa, Joaquin de, 163

Multidisciplinary Research Center in Social Systems, 131
Muñóz, Rodrigo, 89
Mutilation, punitive and self-, 5, 23, 25, 27
Mutis, José Celestino, 115, 116, 118, 119, 121, 125, 126

Narváez, Panfilo de, 89
National Autonomous University of Mexico, School of Medicine, 94-95
Natural History of Cayus Plinius the Second, 126
Navarro, Jaime, 116
New Christians, in Brazil, 110-11
Nieves, Fray Luis, 117
Nobrega, Manoel da, 109
Noronha, Fernando de, 110

Obras Completas de Andrés Bello, 165
Obregón, Alvaro, 95
Observations (Hawkins), 135
obstetrics and surgery, pre-Columbian, 8-9
Ocaranza, Fernando, 7, 96
Office of Royal Physicians, Mexico, 91-92
Ola, Nicolas Méndez de, 91
Olaeta, Méndez de, 91
Olano, G., 7
Opera Medicinalia (Bravo), 90
Operations of Surgery (Heister), 123
Oquendo, Don Antonio de, 133
Ordenanzas para el Buen Gobierno de la Armada Real del Mar Oceano, 136
Ortega, Francisco, 95
Ortíz, Geronimo de, 91
Osorio, Fernández, 91

paccarina, 46
Paiva, Manuel Joaquim Henriques de, 107

Panamerican Federation of Associations of Medical Schools, 131
Parano, Juan Francisco, 114
Paredes, Conde de, 91
passion flower, 72
pathology and diagnosis, pre-Columbia, 7-8
Paul III, Pope, 124
Pavón, José, 126
Pelaez, García, 75
Penalver, José Antonio, 118
Penheiro Morão, Simão, 106
Pequena história da medicína Brasileira (Santos Filho), 108
Peru
  attitudes toward disease in, 44-47
  cancer in, 21-22
  colonial medical education, 124
  congenital malformations, 27-28
  dental problems, 36
  diagnosis, 51-52
  disorders of bone, 18-19
  endocrinological disorders, 27
  eye disorders, 35-36
  fevers, 20-21
  god-germ concept, 50-51
  making war in, 44
  mental functions, 36-39
  mental illness, 39-43
  mercury in, 31-32
  mutual aid in, 43-44
  Peruvian verruga in, 30, 32
  spongy hyperostosis in, 33
  syphilis in, 22-23
  transmission of disease in, 47-50
  tuberculosis in, 28-30
  uta in 23-27
  vitamin C deficiency in, 35
Peruvian verruga
  in ancient Peru, 30, 32
  and Trans-Andean Railroad, 47
Philip II, 90, 106
Philip III, 89

Philip IV, 114, 125
Pires de Lim, Americo, 135
Piso, Willem, 105, 106
Pizarro, Pedro, 23, 32
Place, Nature and Properties of the City of Mexico. Rains and Winds to Which It Is Subject and Climates of the Year (Cisneros), 91
Plantae Novae Hispaniae (Sessé and Mocino), 127
Plascencia, Juan de, 89
Ponta Delgada Public Library, 132
Ponte, Gabriel, 147, 149, 163
Popul Vuh, 55
Pozo, Carlos del, 153, 156-57
pre-Columbia medicine, 1-3
  anatomical knowledge, 7
  and cultural trends, 4-6
  autochthonous and epidemic diseases, 9-12
  and culture, 4-6
  dynamic history, 3
  and ecology, 3-4
  legacy, 14
  pathology and diagnosis, 7-8
  profession, 6-7
  surgery and obstetrics, 8-9
  therapeutics and psychotherapy, 12-14
preventive medicine and public health, teaching, 129-30
Principles of Surgery (Boerhaave), 123
prickly pear, as Mayan food, 72
Principia Medicinae, Epitome et Tortius Humani Corporis Fabrica (Osorio), 91
The Prognostics (Hippocrates), 89
protein-calorie malnutrition, and Mayan diet, 81
protomedicatus, 125-26
psychotherapy and therapeutics, pre-Columbian, 12-14
public health and preventive medicine, teaching, 129-30

Pyrard de Laval, Françoix, 137

Quesada, F., 7
Quintana, Antonio López, 163

Rada, José F., 94
Recordacion Florida (Fuentes), 61
Recuerdos sobre la Rebelión de Caracas (Díaz), 159
Regimento (Esens), 132-38
Reinhepo, Romão Mōsia, 106
Relación de las Cosas de Yucatán (Landa), 59
religion, pre-Columbia, 4-5
research
  community, 130
  scientific, Brazil, 104
Resource Center for Education and Teaching, 131
respiratory system disorders, ancient Peru, 28-30
Restrepo, José Manuel, 126
Rivas, Luis, 147, 165
Rockefeller Foundation, 129
Royal College of Surgeons, Mexico, 92-93
Royal Hospital (Goa), 137
Royal Pontifical University of Mexico, 89, 124
Royal University of San Felipe, 125
Rubiales, Manuel de, 116, 117
Ruiz, Hipólito, 126
Ruiz Moreno, Aníbal, 145

Sahagún, B. de, 7
  on Aztec physicians, 6
Saint Thomas, University of, 115
Salcedo, Matías del, 90
Salgado, José, 93
Salias, Vicente, 147, 161, 168, 169-70
Salinas y Córdova, B., 33, 35
salt, in Yucatán, 75
Sal y Rosas, F., 39, 41-43

San Carlos de Guatemala, University of, 125
San Celedonio, Buenaventura de, 149
San Fulgencio of Quito, University of, 124
sanitary measures, Brazil, 104
Sanitasis Tuenda (Boerhaave), 122
San Juan de Díos Hospital (Santa Fé de Bogotá), 115
San Marcos, University of (Lima), 124
Santillan, F. de, 23
Saraiva, Mateus, 106
School of Medicine for the District and Territories (Mexico), 94
School of Santa Domingo (Santa Fé de Bogotá), 125
School of Santa Rosa (Caracas), 125
scientific expeditions, Latin America, 126-27
scientific literature, Brazil, 105-06
scientific research, Brazil, 104
Sequin, C.A., 39
self-mutilation, pre-Columbian, 5
Serrano y Rubio, Antonio, 93
Sessé, Martin, 127
sexual practices, pre-Columbian, 5-6
Sexto, Dom João, 109
Sigerist, H.E., 52
Sixtus V, Pope, 124
snow blindness, in ancient Peru, 36
Sosa, Manuel de, 90
Sousa, Tomé de, 99
Souza, Nicholas de, 125
spices, Mayan, 70
spirochetosis, 9
squash, as Mayan food, 69
stimulants, pre-Columbian, 4
Stubel, 27
Summary and Compilation of Surgery with a Method of Bleeding, Very Useful and Beneficial (Lopez), 90
Superior College of Our Lady of the Rosary (Santa Fé de Bogotá), 114, 116, 117, 125

The Surgeon's Mate (Woodall), 134
surgery and obstetrics, pre-Columbian, 8-9
susto (fright), 41-42
syphilis, 9, 22-23, 27

tacuatzín, 63, 65
Tadeo Lozano, Jorge, 126
Taiman, A., 36
Tamariz, Felipe, 147, 148, 161
Tejada, Don Vicente Gil, 121, 123
Tello, Julio C., 18, 22, 23
therapeutics and psychotherapy, pre-Columbian, 12-14
Toltecs, 2
Torres, Cristóbal de, 114, 125
tortillas, 59
Trans-Andean Railroad, 47
Tratado único das Bexigas, e Sarampo (Penheiro Morao), 106
The Treasure of Medicine for Various Diseases (Lopez), 91
trees, as Mayan food source, 60-70
trephining, in ancient Peru, 36, 38
Tromp, M.H., 133
True Surgery, Medicine and Astrology (Barrios), 91
tuberculosis, in ancient Peru, 28-30
turkey, as Mayan food, 63, 65-66
turtles, as Mayan food, 64
typhus, 10

U.S. Unitarian Service Committee, 129
Urieta, Francisco de, 89, 90
Urteaga Ballón, Oscar, 18, 33
Ustáriz, Francisco Javier, 147, 156, 164
uta, in ancient Peru, 23-27

vaccination expedition, *See* Balmis expedition
Valdés, Ulíses, 95
Valdés de Cárcamo, Bernabe, 88
Valdizán, H., 39

Valencia, Martín de, 88
Vargas, Nicolás de, 115
Vargas Uribe, Juan Bautista de, 115, 116
vegetables, Mayan growing and consuming, 69
Venezuela, colonial medical education, 125
　See also Balmis expedition
Vergara, Francisco, 118
Verruga, Peruvian, 30, 32
Vertiz, José M., 95
Vertiz, Viceroy, 125
Vieira, Antonio de, 109
Villanueva, Aquilino, 96
Villar, Pedro del, 94
Vellena, Marqués de, 90
Virchow, Rudolph, 24
Viribus Medicamentorum (Boerhaave), 122
vitamin C deficiency in ancient Peru, 35

war, in ancient Peru, 44

weaning, in pre-Columbian period, 3-4
Weiss, Peter, 18, 23, 33
Williams, H.U., 18, 23
women, Mayan, daily life, 75-77
Woodall, John, 134

Ximénez, Francisco
　on beans, 60, 61
　on chocolate, 74
　on corn, 56, 59
　on game animals in Mayan diet, 65-66
　on fruits, 71-72
　on pumpkins, 69
　on Tabasco pepper, 70

Yahuar Huaccac, Emperor, 35

Zárate, Agustín de, 32
Zárraga, Francisco, 95
Zea, Francisco Antonio, 126
Zerda, Messia de la, 115